The Germ
Survival Guide

The Germ Survival Guide

Kenneth A. Bock, M.D.
Steven J. Bock, M.D.
Nancy Faass, MSW, MPH

McGraw-Hill
New York Chicago San Francisco Lisbon London Madrid Mexico City Milan
New Delhi San Juan Seoul Singapore Sydney Toronto

The McGraw·Hill Companies

1 2 3 4 5 6 7 8 9 0   DOC/DOC   0 9 8 7 6 5 4 3

ISBN 0-07-140045-1

McGraw-Hill books are available at special quantity discounts to use as premiums and sales promotions, or for use in corporate training programs. For more information, please write to the Director of Special Sales, Professional Publishing, McGraw-Hill, Two Penn Plaza, New York, NY 10121-2298. Or contact your local bookstore.

This book is for educational purposes. It is not intended as a substitute for medical advice. Please consult a qualified health care professional for individual health and medical advice. Neither McGraw-Hill nor the author shall have any responsibility for any adverse effects arising directly or indirectly as a result of the information provided in this book.

 This book is printed on recycled, acid-free paper containing a minimum of 50% recycled, de-inked fiber.

Library of Congress Cataloging-in-Publication Data

Bock, Kenneth, 1953–

   The germ survival guide / Kenneth A. Bock, Steven J. Bock, and Nancy Faass.
   p. cm.
   Includes bibliographical references and index.
   ISBN 0-07-140045-1
     1. Hygiene.   2. Medicine, Preventive.   3. Communicable diseases—Prevention.
4. Drug resistance in microorganisms. I. Bock, Steven J. II. Faass, Nancy. III. Title.
   RA770.5.B63 2003
   613—dc21

                            2002156359

The following authors have generously given permission for use of extended quotations from their copyrighted works. A portion of Chapter 3, as well as Table 3.7, from Omar Amin, Ph.D. Phoenix: Parasitology Center, Inc., 2002. Chapters 4 and 5 and a portion of Chapter 12 from Elson Haas, MD, *The Staying Healthy Shopper's Guide*. Berkeley, CA: Celestial Arts, 1999. Original research in Chapter 9 courtesy of K. A. Reynolds, P. M. Watt, D. I. Kennedy, and C. P. Gerba. Occurrence of bodily fluid contamination on commonly contacted surfaces and the potential for transfer to the domestic environment. In: *Abstracts of the 100th General Meeting of the American Society for Microbiology*. Los Angeles, CA, May 21–25, 2000. Abstract Q-78. Washington, DC: American Society for Microbiology.

Tables: Information in Table 3.3 courtesy of Diagnos-Techs, Inc., Kent, Washington. Information in Table 4.7 courtesy of Debra Lynn Dadd, *Home, Safe Home* (1996) Tarcher/Putnam, New York. Table 5.3 courtesy Jeffry Anderson, MD. From "What about water?" in *Boosting Immunity*. Len Saputo, MD, and Nancy Faass, eds. Novato, CA: New World Library, 2002. Tables 12.2, 12.3, and 12.4 are reproduced with the permission of Health Press Limited from A. J. Pollard and D. R. Murdoch. *Fast Facts—Travel Medicine*. Oxford: Health Press, 2001.

Contents

1

Outsmarting
the Germs

1

Your Best Defenses

Erin was constantly fatigued and suffered from a range of respiratory problems and sinus infections. Her nine-year-old daughter had severe coughing spells and watery eyes. Tests confirmed her suspicions, revealing construction flaws in her new house and high levels of several molds. Repairs have cost her over $600,000 and there is more yet to be done.

—*San Francisco Chronicle*[1]

Mike played baseball last Saturday and two days later, lay dying at Children's Hospital from what first appeared to be a common flu bug—which turned out to be meningitis.

—*San Francisco Chronicle*[2]

Sarah and Kristin developed skin ulcers after having pedicures in a nail parlor, apparently from a microbe that is cousin to tuberculosis bacteria. They learned that taking antibiotics for months does not always clear the infection. Some of the women who were

3

affected suffered scarring or needed skin grafts . . . esti-mated medical costs for some have exceeded $10,000.
—Adapted, New York Times[3]

Taylor, a seven-year-old cancer patient, celebrated the end of his chemotherapy with an orange juice smoothie. Within a day, he had to be rushed back to the hospital, where it took him four more days to recover. The unpasteurized juice, it turned out, con-tained salmonella.
—New York Times[4]

[On a cruise to Hawaii, Jim] was quarantined in his stateroom . . . and could get food only through room service. . . . Nearly 250 passengers and crew of the cruise ship came down with a gastrointestinal illness during the ship's voyage from Los Angeles to . . . Kauai and Maui. . . . It wasn't known if the ill were suffering from Norwalk or Norwalk-like viruses, which afflicted more than 1500 cruise ship passengers in recent months.[5]
—Adapted, Associated Press[5]

MOST OF US HAVE no memory of life before antibiotics and vaccines. Prior to the twentieth century, the world lived in dread of contagious diseases such as diphtheria, measles, polio, rabies, and smallpox. For the past 60 years, modern medicine has successfully combatted these harmful diseases. Yet worldwide, infectious disease has continued to be the leading cause of early death, accounting for 17 million of nearly 52 million deaths each year.[6] Tuberculosis is the leading cause of these fatalities (4 million), and gastrointestinal infections from microbes like cholera and typhoid are second (3 million). New forms of contagious illness are also on the rise.

We've always been engaged in a life-or-death contest for survival with germs. In the fourteenth century, a third of Europe succumbed to the plague. In the Victorian era, tuberculosis killed one-fourth of all Europeans. At the end of World War I, an estimated 40 million people perished from a flu pandemic in less than a year.[7] According to the International Commission on Hygiene, about half the world's population contracted this influenza. The lightning speed of the disease's course took millions by surprise. And often it was the strongest men and women who perished, with over 80 percent of deaths occurring in people aged 17 to 40.

The widespread success of antibiotics following World War II gave hope of a final end to the tragic problem of infectious disease. Antibiotics provided new options for treating often-fatal conditions, such as cholera, food poisoning, infected wounds, meningitis, pneumonia, tuberculosis, and typhoid fever. But the limitations of the "wonder drugs" soon became apparent. In 1946, just 5 years after the introduction of penicillin, doctors discovered a strain of staph bacteria that had become resistant to the drug. This information wasn't widely announced. New and stronger antibiotics were developed. We moved forward with the impression we had won the "war against disease." But the microbes have continued to adapt and mutate, to overcome each new generation of antibiotics.

> *Our anti-microbial drugs have become less effective . . . and experts in infectious diseases are concerned about the possibility of a "post-antibiotic era." At the same time, our ability to detect, contain, and prevent emerging infectious diseases is in jeopardy. . . . We*

> *know we will never conquer infectious diseases. The*
> *question is whether we can control these organisms so*
> *we can co-exist.*
> —Dr. David Satcher, former U.S. Surgeon General[8]

The adaptive capacity of the microbes reflects the amazing power of nature. Equally impressive is the fact that humans and animals can coexist with such powerful forces. However, the remarkable balance that nature has created can be upset. It is unlikely that destroying this balance will occur without negative consequences. Through the use of antibiotics, it appears that we are now able to treat many bacterial infections. However, we are beginning to see the far-reaching impact of this approach and its dangerous effects. It may be that we will need to learn to work with nature by supporting our innate immunity. Prevention is perhaps most consistent with nature's way of keeping us healthy.[9]

What You Can Do About It

Germs are making a comeback—the growing list of drug-resistant bacteria includes toxic *E. coli*, meningitis bacteria, salmonella, staph, strep, and tuberculosis. Although the threat of infectious illness is frightening, there are practical, commonsense steps we all can take. Whenever we avoid illness, it means we have avoided doing battle with germs—completely sidestepping the need for medication or the potential of an infection that might be resistant to treatment. It also means less time lost from work, fewer medical bills, and better quality of life. By becoming informed and proactive, we can protect ourselves and our families more effectively. In the war against disease, information is one of our best defenses.

1. Strengthen your immunity. Build your resistance. No matter who you are—working parent, growing child, busy professional, or retiree—your immune system is your primary defense against illness. Without immune defenses, even the most powerful drugs cannot fully protect us, as we've learned from the AIDS epidemic. The new research can be used to focus our efforts on the most practical strategies for building strong immunity. (For a quick review of immune building, see Chapter 2.)

- For example, we all realize that sleep is important to health. Yet about 70 percent of Americans get less than 8 hours of sleep a night.[10] A survey by the American Cancer Society of more than 1 million people found what we all have suspected—8 hours seems to be the magic number to maintain good health.[11]

2. Reduce your exposure. What action steps do you need to take to avoid contagion? It's easier to be proactive when you know what to do. Prevention may not be exciting, but it's way ahead of all the other strategies available to us. We'll alert you to situations that expose you to risk (and suggest steps you can take to cut your risk). For example:

- Your kitchen sponge has more bacteria than any other object in your home.
- Your mattress may contain more mold than your bathroom.
- City tap water has been found to contain bad bugs such as giardia, cryptosporidium, and various bacteria.
- *E. coli* can be transmitted by petting zoo animals, and salmonella can be transmitted by handling turtles and baby chicks.

- In terms of public places, playgrounds have more
  germs than pay phones or park benches.

3. Use natural medicine at home. Get rid of colds at the
first sign of a sniffle when vitamins, herbs, and homeopathic
remedies work the best.
- Natural medicine offers a range of options for fighting
  common viral infections such as colds or mild flu in
  the early stages. We'll review the latest research on the
  effectiveness of natural remedies.
- It is also important to know when to stop self-treating
  and go to see the doctor. The risk of serious illnesses
  such as meningitis makes this a very real concern.

4. Use antibiotics wisely. Ask your doctor for antibiotics
only when you really need them. Colds and flu are caused by
viruses, against which antibiotics have no effect. Understanding
the most intelligent use of medication can help us save them
for when we need them most. Remember, the doctor is less
likely to prescribe unnecessary medication if we don't ask for it.

**5. Use integrative medicine—the best of mainstream
medicine and complementary and alternative therapies—
when you want additional options.** The combination of
mainstream medicine and complementary therapies gives you
the best of both worlds. It's helpful to have a range of strategies.
An integrative physician can guide you in the skilled use of vitamins and herbs and when you need an antibiotic, he or she can
prescribe that as well.

6. Support public health. Our quality of life is in large
part a reflection of federal and municipal efforts to maintain

clean water and air in order to provide good sanitation and control infectious disease.

The Global Problem of Infectious Illness

The recent increase in infectious illness is driven by enormous global changes. Due to international travel, transport, migration, and immigration, it is now possible to be exposed to germs from anywhere in the world. When we travel, we may come in contact with exotic microbes that have emerged from the destruction of the rain forests or the breakdown of other ecosystems. Since millions of people travel internationally each year, including millions of Americans, the potential for germ exchange is tremendous. In the United States, almost half our food is shipped in from overseas. At a time when exposure is increasing, our immune systems may be less up to the job. Most of us have some degree of constant exposure to toxic chemicals, including petroleum products, pesticides, and industrial wastes. And if we live or work in a city, as more than 90 percent of us do, we also experience increased exposure to germs in our overcrowded megacities. Modern living comes at a price, reflected in the escalation of contagious illness.

Forty years ago, the consensus was that infectious disease was a thing of the past—that we were no longer vulnerable to epidemics. A researcher at the Centers for Disease Control (CDC) points out, "Changes in the environment, climate, technology, land use, human behavior, and demographics all converge to favor the emergence of infectious diseases. . . . Today's massive movement of humans and materials sets the stage for mixing diverse genetic pools [of microbes] . . . at rates and in combinations previously unknown."[12] An expert panel at the National Institute of Medicine[13] has defined some of the major causes:

- The overuse of antibiotics
- The decline of public health
- Changes in the way our food is produced
- World travel and trade
- Overpopulation and the density of our cities
- Megacities in less developed nations and tropical areas
- Changes in the environment
- Human destruction of the tropical rain forests
- Global warming
- Changes in our lifestyle
- The adaptability of the microbes

Emerging Issues

Over the past 20 years, every nation has experienced the emergence of new forms of infectious disease. The problems are varied and complex:

- **Drug-resistant microbes.** Resistant infections have been an emerging public health problem since 1985. By 1993, the records show that more than 70,000 Americans were dying from drug-resistant infections acquired in hospitals. In the year 2000, more than 109,000 Americans died of hospital-acquired infections.[14] The CDC estimates that in 1995 there were approximately 279,000 cases of these drug-resistant infections.[15] In 2001, there were reports that the HIV virus had mutated beyond the latest forms of drug therapy.

- **Old diseases.** Illnesses that were once thought to be under control have developed drug-resistant strains. Drug-resistant tuberculosis is a case in point. About 20,000 new cases are identified each year. Drug-resistant strains of tuberculosis are difficult to treat and are most prevalent in prisons, homeless shelters, and other institutional settings. The CDC labels these old diseases *reemerging infectious diseases*. In addition to tuberculosis the most dangerous include new types of malaria, gonorrhea, and cholera. These strains develop naturally as the microbes continually adapt to challenges in their environment, such as antibiotics. Occasionally, spontaneous changes occur within the microbes' genetic makeup, enabling them to survive more efficiently—these are considered mutations. The new, more aggressive strains are familiar microbes that have mutated.

- **New microbes.** New sources of infection are regarded as *emerging infectious diseases*—and they are becoming more commonplace. They often occur as a result of natural genetic changes in existing microbes. At least 30 new disease-causing agents have been discovered by researchers during the past two decades—including AIDS, Legionnaires' disease, and Lyme disease, as well as the Ebola, Marburg, and West Nile viruses. New sources of infection continue to be identified. They include hepatitis D and herpes 6A and 6B. Herpes 6A can be big trouble—apparently it is a major cause of chronic fatigue syndrome, fibromyalgia, and other conditions. It works by shutting down the immune function, thus opening the door for other viruses such as Epstein-Barr (which causes mononucleosis) and cytomegalovirus, associated with AIDS.

- **Supergerms.** The most frightening and potentially threatening class of microbe is the supergerm—strains of bacteria and viruses that can cause immediate, intense symptoms that are often fatal. Many are exotic rain forest viruses that are being unearthed as the tropical jungles are destroyed. Emerging supergerms include Ebola, Lassa fever, Marburg hantavirus, and dengue fever. The plague is another present-day example. Luckily only a few cases turn up each year. For example, it was recently disturbed from wilderness areas in the Arizona desert during the construction of new housing developments.

AIDS is the ultimate supergerm. Like many of these pathogens, it may have begun in the African rain forests. The first major outbreak in the United States was discovered in 1981. Although the AIDS epidemic was thought to be slowing in the United States, it still accounts for almost 60,000 new cases here every year and 5.8 million new cases worldwide.[16] In some segments of the U.S. population, it is the leading cause of death.[17] The tricky part about all these diseases is their persistence.

■ **Germs transmitted by animals.** Some supergerms have migrated from animals to people, causing illnesses described as zoonotic infections. Many common diseases initially infected only animals. Lethal diseases that have recently been identified in human hosts include mad cow disease from prions in cattle, as well as the highly virulent Asian bird flu, which is caused by a virus. Cats are believed to be a primary carrier of *Heliobacter pylori*, the bacteria that cause ulcers.

■ **Germ warfare.** The Centers for Disease Control and Prevention has identified the most likely weapons of bioterrorism. The threat of contagious illness comes primarily from harmful bacteria and viruses. Bacterial threats include anthrax, botulism toxins, plague, and tularemia. Smallpox could potentially be revived—a disease almost totally eradicated from the Western Hemisphere.

■ **New links between infection and illness.** Researchers have found startling evidence that microbes play a major role in the development of diseases not previously linked to infection, such as cancer and heart disease. Science now defines an entire class of viruses as cancer-causing (oncogenic) viruses. Human papilloma virus is reported to cause cervical cancer in about 8 out of every 10 cases.[18] A new vaccine for the prevention of human papilloma virus has recently been released. Kaposi's sarcoma, caused by a virus, results in a highly destructive type of skin cancer associated with AIDS. A form of chlamydia bacteria has been linked to heart disease, according to the *Journal of the American Medical Association*.[19] We also now know from research that ulcers are often caused by the bacteria *H. pylori*. What we hear about less frequently is that a significant percentage of people with *H. pylori* infections eventually develop stomach cancer or other degenerative diseases.[20] Although the problems of infectious disease are just now gaining a high profile in the media, the CDC has been educating people about reemerging diseases and drug-resistant microbes for over a decade.

The CDC: Our Best Hope

The Centers for Disease Control may be our best hope. It stands unparalleled in the world of science—a huge global network that defends us against disease. The CDC was founded to track infections and diseases. Its job is to identify outbreaks and take swift action to prevent epidemics. To carry out this mission, the CDC works with health departments in every major city, all 50 states, and most countries, through a staff of more than 7000.

The CDC's disease chasers are epidemiologists—scientific sleuths who unravel the mysteries of contagion, from Ebola in Zaire to cryptosporidium in Milwaukee. These disease fighters are experts allied with the World Health Organization and specialists on all continents. They have virtually pushed smallpox into extinction. They also monitor trends, like the dramatic decrease in polio cases with the success of the Salk and Sabin vaccines. And they track the reemergence of diseases such as tuberculosis. Every week, they report data on nationwide trends in more than 50 contagious illnesses based on information from doctors and public health departments across the country.

The CDC and the World Health Organization work together to monitor the rise and fall of disease across the planet. They're watching the evidence of an invisible ecology, the world of microbes. We coexist with these vast species. We all occupy the same space. And although we can't see them and we don't usually think about them, they ultimately affect all our lives.

Why Worry?

Researchers at the CDC try to second-guess global shifts in these huge invisible populations. The researchers' perspective is sobering: In 1992, 13,300 hospital patients died of infections that resisted every drug doctors tried. In 1993, the number jumped fivefold to some 80,000 Americans dying as the result of hospital-acquired antibiotic-resistant infections.[21] By the year 2000, that number had increased to more than 100,000.[22]

"What scares the people of the CDC even more than exotic diseases are the mundane microbes, once easily quashed with antibiotics, that have started defeating even the most powerful drugs," explains Dr. Claire Broome, former deputy director of the CDC.[23]

These are issues that potentially affect us all. One way to deal with them is to educate ourselves about what we can do to minimize our risk and the risk to our children. It's important to be honest with ourselves about the extent of our control over infectious disease. Some infections can be turned around with just a few doses of vitamin C or herbs. Others require drugs—sometimes very strong drugs. But in cases such as AIDS, we have fewer defenses against the microbes. Prevention is still one of our best strategies.

Antibiotics: Too Much of a Good Thing?

[Tom] was in his 70s when he contracted his last kidney infection. He was sent to a nearby suburban hospital. Years of battling kidney disease had weakened his immune system and the infection developed rapidly.

No one knows how the new strain of staph got into the intensive care unit. Doctors in the hospital had carefully restricted the use of their most powerful antibiotics and isolated their sickest patients. Medical personnel had been instructed repeatedly in hygiene and hand washing.

But the strain of staph—Staphylococcus aureus —that [Tom] contracted that day was no ordinary microbe. It happened to be drug-resistant, able to withstand even vancomycin, the antibiotic known as "the silver bullet." Without the protection of the drug, his immune system was overwhelmed by the bacteria and he died.

—Associated Press[24]

In the year 2001, hospital-acquired infections were the fourth leading cause of death in the United States. These infections included antibiotic-resistant strains of staph, like Tom's, that cause toxic shock syndrome. Others were strep infections, including mutant strep that can become flesh-eating bacteria— necrotizing fasciitis.

These are global problems, and they're on the rise:

- In Thailand, *Campylobacter*—which can cause acute gastrointestinal symptoms—tested as completely treatable with ciprofloxacin in 1991. Just 4 years later, 84 percent of the samples were drug-resistant.[25]
- In Iceland, penicillin-resistant strep—the type that can cause pneumonia and meningitis—increased by 8 times in just 3 years. Samples were 2 percent resistant in 1989 and 17 percent in 1992.[26]
- In Holland, drug-resistant *H. pylori*—the bacteria that can cause ulcers and sometimes stomach cancer—increased fourfold from 7 percent in 1993 to 32 percent in 1996.[27]
- In the United States, in 1987, the CDC found no drug-resistant bacteria in a review of test results from more than 6700 lab samples. In samples from 1992, 1 percent were drug-resistant. By 1994, more than 3 percent of the bacteria were totally drug resistant. Now almost 300,000 cases of drug-resistant infection, out of 2 million hospital infections, are reported annually.[28,29]

Too Much, Too Often?

The amount of antibiotics we use is mind-boggling:

- Over 34 million pounds of penicillin are produced and consumed worldwide every year. And that's just penicillin.
- More than 83 million pounds of antibacterial drugs were produced in the United States in 1994, with 40 percent intended for the livestock and poultry industries.

All these drugs are put to use. In 1996, American doctors wrote 133 million patient prescriptions for antibiotics. Of these, an estimated 12 million were for respiratory infections. Yet the vast majority of these infections—colds, flu, and bronchitis—are caused by viruses. Antibiotics have virtually no effect on viruses and are only used to prevent secondary infections from bacteria. New guidelines for antibiotic use have been developed by the Centers for Disease Control. In response, research suggests that antibiotic prescribing is being curtailed by physicians.[30]

Problems of overuse lie with both patients and physicians. Patients sometimes pressure their doctors for antibiotics so they can get back to work. They feel they need instant solutions. Each individual situation ultimately contributes to the growing threat of antibiotic resistance. (See Table 1.1 for more information on drug-resistant microbes.) In response to these issues, the CDC has revised the guidelines for the use of antibiotics.

Antibiotics Down on the Farm

Another major problem with antibiotic overuse occurs in the livestock industry. Most of us haven't realized until recently that every year, millions of tons of antibiotics are used worldwide in raising cattle, sheep, and poultry, mainly as an additive in feed. The Union of Concerned Scientists reports that by the late 1990s more than 25 million pounds were given to livestock annually, whereas only 3 million pounds were used by humans.[31]

Why would cost-conscious farmers and ranchers spend such a large sum of money in raising animals? They consider it a profitable investment and money well spent to prevent disease among their livestock. A sick or dead animal represents a business loss. Too many losses and the farm or ranch is out of business.

Table 1.1   The 10 Top Drug-Resistant Microbes

Microbes/ Reports of resistance	Diseases caused	Examples of drugs resisted
GI bacteria: *Enterobacteriaceae;* 15,726 articles on enterobacter drug resistance	Generalized infections, pneumonia, urinary tract, and surgical wound infections	Ampicillin and penicillin, cephalosporins, chloramphenicol, imipenem, kanamycin, sulfa drugs, tetracycline, trimethoprim
Staph: *Staphylococcus aureus;* 8323 articles	Generalized bacterial infections, pneumonia, surgical wound infections	Chloramphericol, ciprofloxacin, erythromycin, gentamycin, penicillin, rifampicin, tetracycline, trimethoprrim, vancomycin
Pseudomonas aeruginosa 4224 articles	Generalized bacterial infections, pneumonia, urinary tract infections	Chloramphenicol, ciprofloxacin, imipenem, kanamycine, sulfa drugs, tetracycline, trimethroprim
Strep: *Streptococcus pneumoniae;* 3493 articles	Meningitis, pneumonia	Chloramphenicol, ciprofloxacin, erythromycin, penicillin, streptomycin, tetracycline, trimethroprim, vancomycin
GI bacteria: *Enterococcus;* 2954 articles	Generalized infections, urinary tract, and surgical wound infections	Ampicillin and penicillin, ciprofloxacin, kanamycin, tetracycline, vancomycin
Malaria: *Plasmodium falciparum;* 2368 articles	A parasitic infection of the bloodstream	Amodiaquine, artesunate, chloroquine, melfloquine, pyrimethamine, sulfadoxine
Haemphilus influenzae; 1961 articles	Blocked airway, ear and sinus infections, meningitis, pneumonia	Ampicillin and penicillin, chloramphenicol, erythromycin, tetracycline, trimethroprim

Table 1.1 (continued)

Microbes/ Reports of resistance	Diseases caused	Examples of drugs resisted
M. tuberculosis; 2682 articles	Tuberculosis	Ethambutol, isoniazid, pyrazinamide, rifampicin, streptomycin
N. gonorrhoeae; 1500 articles	Gonorrhea	Ciprofloxacin, penicillin, spectinomycin, sulfa drugs, tetracycline
Yeast: Candida albicans; 1408 articles	Fungal overgrowth in the digestive tract, urinary tract, or vagina, systemic infections in immune compromised patients	Amphotericin, fluconazole, flucytosine, itraconazole, nystatin

SOURCE: Content drawn from the Medline data base of the National Library of Medicine. Web site: www.ncbi.nlm.nih.gov/PubMed/.

Antibiotics provide other major benefits to the bottom line. We've heard about the use of growth hormones in raising beef and poultry, but *antibiotic use* is another way to increase growth in livestock. In fact, antibacterial drugs are so often included in feed for this purpose, they can be purchased for animal use without a prescription. The drugs improve the marbling and marketability of meat in beef, hogs, and sheep. Antibiotics also reduce the incidence of "shipping fever syndrome," a disease often contracted by animals during the stress of transport to market. *The Stockman's Handbook,* a popular guide for ranchers, says, "Antibiotics increase weight gain in steers, heifers, and calves by 6% daily while reducing feed requirements by 4%."[32]

That's why antibiotics play such an important part in today's farm economics. The drugs are added in low doses to the *daily* feed of poultry and livestock and into the pond water of farm-raised fish. The good news is that the animals grow faster, get bigger quicker, and go to market earlier, so fewer are lost to disease. The bad news is that antibiotics accumulate in their tissues and remain there, even after slaughter and processing.

We're at the Top of the Food Chain

When we eat chicken, beef, or fish from our local supermarket, we're often consuming antibiotics as well. The drug residues circulate through our bodies and accumulate in our tissues.

Continuous exposure to antibiotics in our food can destroy some of the natural bacteria in our own digestive tracts. We also consume some drug-resistant bacteria in the poultry and meat we eat. We know some of those bacteria are already drug-resistant because they have survived the daily antibiotic dosing of the animal.

These antibacterial medications also find their way into our soil and water. While some break down rapidly, others remain in their active form indefinitely. For example, when antibiotics are used in fish farming, reports suggest that 70 to 80 percent of these drugs end up in the environment.[33]

Although the government regularly tests samples of produce and soil for pesticides, there is currently no testing program in agriculture for either drug residues or resistant bacteria. It's important to note that the incidence of food poisoning in humans has greatly increased since the introduction of antibiotics into animal feed—particularly cases of salmonella (from eggs and poultry products) and *E. coli* (from beef). Most Americans have been unaware of these facts until they were reported in recent congressional testimony.[34]

2

Six Strategies Against Germs

1. Strengthening Your Immunity

What you do can have a profound impact on whether you get sick, how long you're sick, and how seriously ill you become. Research over the past 20 years suggests that a healthy lifestyle, good nutrition, and the use of supplements can provide protective effects. For example, researchers have been able to show the effects of lifestyle on immunity by measuring the vitality of the immune system through markers such as T-cell levels. As a result, it is now possible to determine the immune response to sleep, different types of exercise, nutrients, and other factors. This information can be translated into practical steps anyone can take to strengthen immunity.

We can no longer assume that colds and flu are always harmless or that infectious illness is always self-limiting. New information suggests that common viral infections like colds can sometimes leave us open to more serious conditions, such as debilitating flu, pneumonia, or even meningitis, if they deplete our immunity. In a recent outbreak of cryptosporidium in Canada, health authorities indicated that most people who suffered the flu-like illness would probably recover within 2 weeks, but that the microbe could be deadly to people with immune deficiencies.[1] Understanding the realities of susceptibility, exposure, and immunity can make an important difference to your health.

Building the Foundation for Strong Immunity

Your immune system is your first line of defense against all types of infectious agents, from the viruses that cause the common cold to the bacteria responsible for food poisoning. These efforts can be surprisingly simple.

Your perspective is an important part of the equation. For example, many people find it difficult to change their eating habits because they think they're going to have to "give things up," and feel deprived. Yet most people who eat organic or natural foods find that they've never eaten better in their lives. Changing eating habits is about discovering delicious new foods and cuisine, learning new ways to prepare some old favorites, and, as a special bonus, achieving better health. Key strategies for building strong immunity include:

- Getting plenty of sleep
- Drinking pure water
- Maintaining a realistic exercise program
- Detoxifying your body
- Eating a good diet
- Managing stress

Promoting Good Immunity through Balance

Balance is another essential aspect of strong immunity. Good immunity is not just a matter of boosting the immune system or encouraging it to work even harder. This creates the danger of immune overreactivity, which can result in allergies and autoimmune diseases. Balance in the immune system is the quintessential example of balance in the body and can be compared to balanced function in the nervous system. Within the nervous system, there needs to be a balance between the activity of the neurons and the calming influences that inhibit and quiet the system. When there is too much activity—too many neurons firing—symptoms such as hyperactivity, spasms, or even a seizure can result. The nervous system and immune function are the two most complex systems in the body, and balance is crucial to both.

Clearly, we all want to have a strong immune system to deal with the many insults to which we're exposed—infections, chemicals, and heavy metals. We know that heavy metals such as mercury and lead tend to skew the immune system to a reactive mode in which it produces too much defensive artillery (antibodies) and fewer protective T cells. We are seeing more and more autoimmune conditions, perhaps due in part to these toxic exposures and the loss of balance within the immune system. Restoring balance is a crucial aspect of good health.

At least 60 percent of us carry staph and strep bacteria in our bodies at any one time. If you carry a bug like staph, but keep it contained, as most of us do, that reflects healthy immune function. It's not that we're not exposed to germs—we all have bacteria in our digestive tracts and on our skin. Rather, good health comes back to the question of balance. You don't want to be exposed to an overwhelming number of bugs, so minimizing your exposure is an intelligent strategy. When you limit your exposure to germs, you are more likely to keep the challenge at a level your immune system can handle. You also want your immune system to be effective and able to keep microbes in check.

Nobody loves you more than your own immune system. When it is working correctly, it fights countless battles every day, large and small, to keep you healthy—whether you cooperate or not. Imagine how powerful your immune system will be if you provide it with all the nutrients it needs and take steps to protect it from the poisons and assaults of modern life. These are the basic ingredients for a happy, healthy immune system.

2. Minimizing Your Exposure

Minimizing exposure involves a countless number of little decisions that occur from minute to minute. Consider how germs are spread in an imaginary family that is typical of the real world. We know that many germs are transmitted in droplets from coughing and sneezing and also by touching and person-to-person contact. One family member may be coughing and forgets to cover his mouth. Another puts her hand over her mouth, but then touches one of her children. In that case, she has forgotten that her hands are covered with the virus.

To minimize the spread of germs, there are steps we all must take, steps that need to become second nature. For example, it's quite easy to transmit the bad bugs that can inhabit the digestive tract, particularly if someone has an illness or if there's a young child in the family still in diapers. These germs can continue to spread among family members, conveyed by touch or transmitted during food preparation. (This same potential for transmission also occurs in restaurants.) In all these situations, hand washing is essential, because it breaks the cycle of transmission. As physicians, we know that it's necessary to wash our hands between every patient visit. It's a little inconvenient, but it doesn't matter. It has to be done, because we don't want to transmit germs from one patient to another.

When children are sick, it becomes a challenge to practice ideal hygiene. You have contact with their germs in any number of ways, so there's always a chance you can become ill as well. When your spouse has a cold, do you still kiss your spouse? Or do you wait 2 or 3 days until your spouse feels better? This is also a good time to increase your intake of protective supplements. These are basic behaviors we can build into our lifestyle.

What happens when a family get-together is scheduled and one of the cousins comes down with a bad cold? Do you bring your child, although you know your child and the cousin will spend a lot of time together? Or do you postpone the visit for a few days so you can diminish your child's exposure? What constitutes a healthy, balanced lifestyle? These are basic human issues that have not only health implications but also social ramifications. Such issues need to be dealt with on an individual basis in each family. These questions of balance are profound because they extend from microscopic exposures to the broadest issues in our lives.

3. Nipping Infections in the Bud

Whenever we can shorten the course of illness, we conserve valuable immune resources. We practice this approach personally, and we teach it to our patients. As physicians, there is no way we can avoid germs. Kids cough and sneeze; patients need to have throat cultures taken—by definition, our job is to be around people who are ill.

We must make a greater effort to stay healthy—to eat a good diet, get regular exercise, and take supplements that provide immune support, including vitamin C, transfer factor, and herbs. Transfer factors are the microscopic blueprints our immune systems rely on to recognize and combat germs. When we experience a greater exposure, or feel the early symptoms of a viral infection, that's the time to increase from maintenance doses to more therapeutic doses. A number of effective strategies increase immune protection. We may triple the intake of vitamin C and the doses of Transfer Factor, an immune-supportive product. This is also the time to take antiviral herbs such as echinacea and goldenseal. We may opt to take immune enhancers, like those found in Chinese mushrooms. The key is to be aware of what you've been exposed to and how your body responds. You want to be proactive right then to step up the immune support when it will make a difference. Once you sense that you have successfully fought off the infection, you can gradually return to the maintenance level of your supplements.

Personally, we find this approach to be extremely effective. We often see others around us becoming ill while we manage to stay well, using these strategies. We also see the benefits of this approach in our patients. For example, we've observed major changes in the health of the asthmatic children in our practice, who often come to us with a history of severe bronchitis, frequent asthma attacks, and sinus infections. Once they begin taking supplements, and their exposure to environmental and food allergies is decreased, their infections become less frequent, briefer, and less intense. In fact, we see this almost universally among our patients.

4. Using Vaccinations and Antibiotics Wisely

Vaccinations

Vaccinations play an important role in the public's health. They prevent illnesses and prevent epidemics. Vaccinations have decreased the incidence of many infectious diseases, particularly devastating viruses such as polio and smallpox.

How do immunizations work? During active immunization, the person to be protected is injected with a killed or altered version of a particular infectious microbe. The immune system generates memory cells against the microbe. These cells memorize and record the profile of the infectious agent. This means that the next time this microorganism is encountered, the immune system can respond with an immediate full defense. For example, the next time there's exposure to measles or poliovirus, the memory cells can quickly call up an effective immune response against that particular virus.

For the vast majority of people, this provides protection against diseases that are potentially life-threatening. However, individuals who have a dysfunctional immune system may experience increased health concerns due to vaccines. In a susceptible individual, vaccines can skew the balance of the immune system. This is particularly true of newborns and certain children, due to the immaturity of their immune systems and their increased vulnerability. A highly sensitive child can become prone to immune-related disorders such as allergies, asthma, ear infections, or eczema.

In our work with autistic children, we have seen a link between the use of certain vaccines and the development of immune dysfunction. Some vaccines contain mercury, in an additive called thimerasol. Although this additive has recently been taken off the market, some vaccines containing thimerasol are still in use. There is real concern that thimerasol can initiate a process that may be skewing the immune system into a reactive mode of antibody overproduction and impaired T-cell function. At a very young age, American children once received multiple vaccinations, a number of which contained mercury. It is possible that these vaccines contributed to the epidemic of autism we are now seeing and also possibly to the tremendous increase in attention deficit hyperactivity disorder.

Mercury is a known toxin that has been banned from many other products—for example, mercury thermometers are no longer available, Mercurochrome no longer contains mercury, and mercury-containing eyedrops are no longer marketed. Even after these products were taken off the market, the vaccines intended for our youngest children still contained mercury—in fact, until recently, pediatricians were giving these vaccines to newborns 1 day old.

This issue is being brought to the forefront in Congress, and to date, the pharmaceutical companies have taken thimerasol out of the vaccinations. This will make the vaccines safer for children. Safety is the primary concern. We are not antivaccination—rather we are pro safe vaccinations.

Antibiotics

We know that antibiotics have expanded our ability to fight infectious bacteria beyond anyone's expectation. Some antibiotics are bacteriocidal, meaning they kill bacteria outright. Others are bacteriostatic, meaning they prevent the bacteria from growing or multiplying. Antibiotics do not harm normal cells, and each antibiotic is effective only against specific types of bacteria. Yet even if you're on antibiotics, your immune system still has to mop up and filter out the debris caused by an infection. When taking antibiotics, there are a few key points to remember:

- **Antibiotics are effective only against bacteria.** If you have a sore throat caused by a virus, although it may look and feel like strep throat (caused by streptococcus bacteria), an antibiotic won't help. On the other hand, if you have a strep infection, an antibiotic is usually the most effective medication.

- **Always take the entire course of the antibiotic.** Short-term use of antibiotics can kill off the less resistant bacteria while the stronger ones survive. If they are allowed to multiply, you'll have a tougher infection to beat. This is why your doctor will insist that you take an antibiotic for the entire recommended time.

- **Request antibiotics only when you really need them.** Ask your doctor if you have a bacterial infection. You don't want to put pressure on your doctor to give you antibiotics unless he or she definitely feels you have a bacterial infection.

- **Take yogurt or acidophilus after using antibiotics.** Our natural digestive flora provide an important line of defense against harmful microbes and play a role in good immune function. We recommend that you take a bottle of acidophilus — probiotics — during and after any course of antibiotics. This can help to restore your beneficial digestive flora. More than 1000 articles in the medical literature demonstrate the importance of maintaining good flora.

- **Minimize the amount of antibiotics you consume in your daily diet.** If you eat meat or fish, select organic meat or fish whenever possible. By definition, this is poultry, beef, lamb, pork, and fish raised without the use of antibiotics. Consider increasing your use of other protein sources such as soy and nuts, as well as eggs and organic dairy products. Decreasing your intake of animal protein tends to lower your levels of antibiotics, resistant bacteria, and toxins.

■ **You can also support new laws to control the use of antibiotics in raising animals.** A number of countries, including New Zealand, have already taken action and outlawed the sub-therapeutic use of antibiotics in farm animals. (See the Resources section at the back of the book for additional information.)

5. Using Integrative Medicine When You Want Additional Options

Integrative medicine is a unifying approach to health care. It combines the best of Western medicine with new scientific research and proven complementary therapies, such as nutrition, herbal therapy, acupuncture, massage and bodywork, homeopathy, chiropractic, and stress management. This provides doctors with additional effective treatments, expanding the options for preventing and treating illness. Integrative medicine also includes strategies you can use at home to protect yourself and your family. Integrative medicine is not "alternative" or "complementary" medicine—rather it is *good* comprehensive medicine.

The history of our practice reflects the benefits of combining both approaches. In 1983, we opened the Rhinebeck Health Center in Upstate New York. We immediately sought admitting privileges to the local hospital and made the effort to become an integral part of the medical community in Rhinebeck. We developed a reputation as rather conservative integrative physicians. It did not take long to build up a busy practice. The health center clearly filled a need. We emphasized natural, noninvasive, nontoxic treatments as much as possible, and we went to great lengths to discover underlying illnesses or conditions that had previously eluded detection.

Medicine is a partnership. Listening is the key. What is the patient looking for? Is there another or more serious condition underlying the illness? What forms of treatment will be of greatest benefit to the patient—treatment that the patient can feel comfortable with. Not everyone who comes into our office is ready to use an inhaler or, on the other hand, is interested in taking Chinese herbs. So we take treatment in stages, building mutual trust. It is senseless for us to give recommendations if a patient is not comfortable with them and is not going to follow them. Patient compliance is an essential key to healing, but patient compliance often begins with flexibility and insight on the part of the physician.

Each human being is unique, physically and spiritually. This is one reason why a "cookie-cutter" approach cannot work for everyone. We closely monitor our patients' responses to treatment, fully aware that what works for one might not work for the next. We consider an individualized approach one of the foundations of good medicine.

At this point in our practice, the patients who find their way to us usually have complex problems that have eluded diagnosis and treatment. Often their immune systems are overburdened. We are happiest when we can solve a medical mystery or progress one step further in the treatment of someone who is ill. In this way, our patients have been our teachers. We find that even with complex conditions, there is often more that can be done, but only if the patient is willing to be open to new possibilities and points of view. Starting to look for the underlying cause of symptoms is like beginning a journey. Sometimes the route is uncertain, but the destination—good health—is always clear. We don't always have the answer, but we continue to push the envelope, looking for new ways to help our patients.

You may be wondering how this perspective relates to a book about germs. Microbiology—the study of microbes and their effects on health—has been an important aspect of mainstream medicine since Leeuwenhoek invented the microscope in the seventeenth century. After 300 years, this field is still a frontier area of medicine, one in which important new information continues to be discovered. Consider the question of antibiotic resistance. The work of the microbiologists has enabled us to track the development of antibiotic resistance over the past 20 years. Similarly, these scientists make possible our understanding of emerging diseases from West Nile virus to Severe Acute Respiratory Syndrome (SARS).

To a certain degree, integrative medicine also has contributions to make in the understanding and treatment of infectious illness. Why? Many of the patients who come to integrative practitioners see us when all else has failed. They usually have complex problems that have eluded diagnosis and treatment. Mainstream medicine has assumed that what we offer is primarily encouragement and hope—also known as the placebo effect. However, another perspective is emerging.

As more sophisticated testing becomes available, it is clear that some of the people we see actually have undiagnosed infectious illness. Almost universally, these are the types of infections that are the most difficult to diagnose and to treat. They include conditions such as Lyme disease (caused by a bacteria that often requires extensive long-term antibiotic treatment); viral illnesses that may underlie certain cases of chronic fatigue syndrome; parasitic infections; and yeast overgrowths (for example, candida infections). In the treatment of these illnesses, we often use antibiotics and other medications. We also recommend good nutrition, supplements, homeopathy, and herbs to support immune function, as well as specific therapies such as acupuncture.

The advantage of integrative medicine is that it doesn't abandon familiar, proven treatments just to promote alternative therapies. The choice of treatment is based on safety, effectiveness, the needs of individual patients, and the requirements of their specific conditions.

6. Supporting Public Health

Many of us have had the impression that the war against disease was won with the invention of antibiotics. In fact, our good health is the result of innovations both in medicine and in public health. Infectious illness has been controlled in industrial nations in part through the great public health reforms that began in the late nineteenth century. These reforms led to the introduction of urban water purification and sewage disposal. For example, in America and England 200 years ago, there were no indoor flush toilets and no sewage disposal. Much of the drinking water was contaminated, and cholera and typhoid spread easily. Now in most industrialized cities, an underground disposal system separates sewage from drinking water. Most cities also provide garbage disposal, street cleaning, rodent control, and toxic waste disposal. The contribution of this public health infrastructure is taken for granted by most of us, until we travel to areas where these amenities are not available.

One of the reasons that we have less infectious illness than our great-grandparents is that we have this infrastructure. Consider all the services provided by the city, state, and federal government that minimize our exposure to infectious microbes in public environments. We have municipal water purification, indoor plumbing, and laws that regulate water and air quality.

Other than climate, this is one of the major differences between industrialized societies and developing nations.

It is in our best interest to support city, state, and federal efforts that maintain our public health infrastructure. Budget cuts in recent years are likely to bring long-term consequences. Get involved in the decisions made in your community regarding important basic issues such as clean air and water. It is important not to take these for granted.

3

The Cast of Characters

Let's consider some of the everyday problems germs can cause, how they do damage, and how we can minimize our exposure to them. Infectious diseases are defined by the Centers for Disease Control as "human illnesses that are caused by microorganisms or their poisonous byproducts." Most sources of infectious illness are microscopic, but include a few other agents of harm, such as larger parasites and the insects that transport disease. Major players include:

- Bacteria
- Viruses
- Protozoa (microscopic parasites)
- Fungi, yeast, and their toxins
- Insect-borne diseases, large parasites, toxic algae, and prions

The CDC tracks the data across the United States on infectious illnesses caused by bacteria and other microbes. These statistics are published weekly, which enables public health officials to follow trends and potential outbreaks. Drawing from the CDC data, we've listed illnesses that are the most frequent or the most serious. It's important to note that the actual number of cases of any given illness is probably quite a bit higher than the numbers reported into the system. For example, in the case of salmonella-related food poisoning, the CDC estimates that the actual incidence is 38 times higher than the number of reports it receives.

Each species or strain has its own life cycle, characteristics, and means of transmission. Microbes may be transmitted in food and water, through the air, through direct contact such as touch, from person to person, and by contact with animals or insects. Here's a brief review of the major microbes and how they cause illness.

Bacteria

Are Ulcers Caused by Stress or Bacteria?

Ulcers used to be considered a condition brought on by stress. But 20 years ago, Dr. Barry Marshall discovered through routine hospital research that ulcers could be caused by the bacteria Helicobacter pylori. He knew that he had identified something important, but he was unable to get the funding he needed to continue further research. Frustrated, he took the do-it-yourself approach and drank a test tube of H. pylori to prove his point. Two weeks later, he developed a full-blown case of stomach ulcers. He got the funding—and the rest is history. Today, antibiotics are prescribed for many cases of ulcers, whenever testing indicates they are caused by bacteria.

Overview

Bacteria are the most abundant form of life on Earth—there are about 4000 known species. Surprisingly, the vast majority of bacteria are harmless. These single-cell organisms are microscopic and invisible to the naked eye. They are related in structure to most other types of microbes—rather than to the plant or animal kingdom.

Beneficial Aspects

Bacteria are essential to many of the processes necessary to life on earth:

- Bacteria that were formerly classified as blue-green algae actually produced much of the oxygen now in the earth's atmosphere.
- Some bacteria "fix nitrogen" in the soil, an essential step that enables plants to create amino acids, the building blocks of protein.
- Other bacteria aid in the creation of humus, the richest kind of soil, which is formed on the forest floor as leaves and organic matter are broken down.
- Bacteria are being used in a variety of human endeavors, from the development of antibiotics and other pharmaceuticals to food technology and the mining industry.
- Within our own bodies, lactobacilli (also found in yogurt) produce lactic acid, which restricts the growth of potentially harmful microbes.

Potential Risks

Bacteria are also the leading cause of human illness, transmitted in a variety of ways. Common bacterial illnesses include food poisoning (for example, E. coli, listeria, and salmonella) and sexually transmitted diseases (such as chlamydia and gonorrhea). Staph and strep bacteria can cause localized infections, particularly in wounds or incisions, and are often implicated in hospital-acquired infections. Airborne bacteria can also be quite formidable—for example, Legionnaires' disease and tuberculosis. (See Table 3.1.)

Bacteria—the Cast of Players

Researchers classify bacteria based on their size, shape, and appearance under the microscope. Bacteria may be spherical (cocci), rod-shaped (bacilli), or spiral-shaped (spirochetes, spirilla, and vibrio). Some have a thick external layer (bacteria

Table 3.1   Bacteria That Can Cause Disease

Airborne bacteria infections	
Tuberculosis	16,377
Whooping cough (pertussis)	7,867
Legionnaires' disease	1,1277
	25,000+ cases yearly
Bacterial food poisoning *(from food and water)*	
Salmonella infections	39,574
Shigella infections	29,922
Hemorrhagic *E. coli* infection	4,528
	More than 70,000 cases
Sexually transmitted diseases *caused by bacteria*	
Chlamydia	700,461
Gonorrhea	358,440
Syphilis, total all stages	5,971
	More than 1 million cases

Source: Data from CDC. Summary of Notifiable Diseases—United States, 2000.
Morbidity and Mortality Weekly Report. 2002, June 14; 49 (53): 1–102.
Web site: www.cdc.gov/mmwr/preview/mmwrhtml/mm4953al.htm.

that can be stained in lab processing—described as gram-positive) and others, a thin outer shell (which does not stain well, termed gram-negative). Many require oxygen to live, just as we do, and are defined as aerobic. Many others are able to survive without oxygen, known as anaerobic. Of these, some can survive in either state, just by "turning their metabolism down" and producing less energy. Surprisingly, more than 98 percent of the bacteria in the digestive tract are anaerobes that survive without oxygen—and therefore rarely appear in a laboratory analysis.

In addition, some bacteria can also assume an inactive spore form when conditions in the environment become inhospitable. The spore functions more like a seed and later becomes active again once the environment is more favorable to survival. These spores can remain dormant for extended periods of time and yet remain viable—capable of regeneration after periods as long as 100 years.

Three categories of bacteria are among the smallest forms of life on earth—chlamydia, mycoplasma, and rickettsia, which live inside the body's cells just as viruses do. (See Table 3.2 for a list of different types of bacteria.) Since they can be harbored within the cell, they tend to cause illnesses that are invasive, lingering, and often difficult to diagnose.

Table 3.2   Types of Bacteria and the Illnesses They Cause

Gram-negative bacteria, by location in the body:
- *Respiratory tract:* Legionella (which causes Legionnaires' disease), meningococcal bacteria (meningitis), pertussis (whooping cough)
- *Intestinal tract*
  - bacteria that cause "dysbiosis" (bacterial overgrowth, potentially chronic conditions)—bacteroides, enterobacter, klebsiella, proteus, pseudomonas

Table 3.2 *(continued)*

- bacteria that cause food poisoning—*E. coli,* salmonella, shigella
- bacteria that cause acute infectious illness—hemorrhagic or toxic forms of *E. coli, Salmonella typhi* (typhoid fever), *Yersinia pestis* (plague)
  - *Elsewhere in the body*
  - bacteria that cause sexually transmitted disease—certain chlamydia, N. gonorrhea, treponema, gardnerella (vaginosis)
  - others: fusobacterium (cause of gum disease); haemophilus (bacterial meningitis), klebsiella and pseudomonas bacteria (can both cause pneumonia)

Families of gram-positive bacteria

- Clostridium, including botulism (colitis, food poisoning, gangrene, tetanus)
- Anthrax and diphtheria (both cause invasive respiratory conditions), listeria (food poisoning)
- Mycobacteria (tuberculosis and leprosy)
- Staphylococcus (abscesses, boils, toxic shock syndrome, wound infections)
- Streptococcus (sore throrat, scarlet fever, heart damage, pneumonia, tooth decay)

Spiral bacteria

- Treponema (syphilis—STD), Borrelia (Lyme disease—tick-borne), campylobacter (can cause colitis and diarrhea), *H. pylori* (causes stomach ulcers); *Vibrio cholerae* (causes cholera)

Exceptionally minute bacteria

- Chlamydia: *Chlamydia trachomatis* (leading STD in United States), *Chlamydia pneumonia* (recently implicated in heart disease), *Chlamydia psittaci* (pneumonia spread by birds, poultry)
- Mycoplasma (one form causes pneumonia; the other is a sexually transmitted disease)
- Rickettsia (tick-borne Rocky Mountain spotted fever and typhus) and ehrlichia (systemic infections)

SOURCE: Information drawn from Peter Q. Warinner, M.D. *Clinical Microbiology Review*. Long Island, NY: Wysteria, 2001.

Chlamydia (a disease caused by a form of bacteria called *Chlamydia trachomatis*) is currently the most prevalent sexually transmitted disease (STD) in the United States, causing over 700,000 new cases each year. Although this condition can be quite treatable, it is often difficult to diagnose. The disease is described as "silent" because many people do not have symptoms. Men tend to be more symptomatic than women. Women who are sexually active and at risk for chlamydia will want to periodically have a pelvic exam or request a culture for lab analysis. Other forms of chlamydia (*Chlamydia pneumoniae*) have been implicated in the development of heart disease and possibly multiple sclerosis.

Mycoplasma are the smallest life-form on earth. Existing entirely without a cell wall, these bacteria operate more like viruses, living inside the cells of their host. As a result, they are impervious to the activity of penicillin, which destroys bacteria by compromising the cell membrane. Mycoplasma have been implicated in Gulf War syndrome, which includes symptoms of chronic fatigue. Persistent bacterial infections caused by mycoplasma have been diagnosed in veterans, particularly those whose immune response was compromised by exposure to the toxic chemicals of the Gulf War environment and possibly the prophylactic vaccinations they received.

Mycobacteria, a family of bacteria that includes tuberculosis and leprosy, is mentioned here to differentiate them from mycoplasma. Mycobacteria tuberculosis is of importance to humanity because of its role as the leading cause of death worldwide due to infectious illness, resulting in 4 million fatalities annually.

Tuberculosis (TB) also deserves scrutiny as slow-growing bacterium, for example when compared with a rapidly dividing bacterium such as strep. TB's long life cycle is one of the reasons it is much less susceptible to antibiotic treatment. Strep, in contrast, is more easily destroyed with antibiotics because there is more frequent opportunity to interrupt its brief life cycle. This makes it possible for the antibiotics to destroy the bacteria during the process of cell division. The tuberculosis bacillus has a life cycle of about 28 days (in contrast to many bacteria with life cycles of about 20 minutes). This means the infection must be treated for a much longer period of time—for months rather than just days or weeks. TB may require a treatment protocol with several antibiotics, taken for 9 to 18 months. The treatment of Lyme disease poses similar problems and may require antibiotics from 4 to 12 weeks or longer, rather than the 3-week treatment that is sometimes utilized.

Gonorrhea is the other most prevalent sexually transmitted disease caused by bacteria, resulting in more than 350,000 reported cases each year. (For additional information on these conditions and others, see Chapter 8 on person-to-person transmission.)

Streptococcal and staphylococcal bacteria are two other families of prevalent microbes we hear about frequently. Strep can cause those severe sore throats that worry every parent. Staph is often associated with infections acquired in the hospital. As we've mentioned, 60 percent of the population or more is estimated to carry these bacteria (usually in the nose and throat area). The fact that our immune systems keep them in check affirms the importance of strong immunity.

Beneficial Bacteria

Our inner ecology also consists of bacteria in the digestive tract—the microflora that include more than 400 species of living bacteria. Among the bacteria, the "friendly flora" play a major role in our digestive process. They include acidophilus, L. bulgaricus, bifidus bacteria, and S. thermophilus, the beneficial bacteria also found in yogurt. These bacteria take part in the manufacture of valuable nutrients such as vitamin K (for clotting), folic acid, and the essential fatty acid butyrate. They also help to keep this inner ecology in balance by producing substances that suppress microbial growth, crowding out harmful microbes, and by maintaining an acidic environment destructive to other less preferred microbes.

Harmless Bacteria That Coexist with Us

Microbes in our bodies that are harmless are described as commensals. In the digestive tract, benign forms of E. coli make up a major portion of the bacteria population. Candida albicans, a form of yeast, is another harmless resident of the digestive tract. If beneficial bacteria are destroyed due to the use of antibiotics, and not replaced, harmless microorganisms can "overgrow" and cause digestive disorders. An overgrowth can also result when infection is present. If the immune system is compromised in any way, it can no longer maintain the balance and keep the bacteria or yeast in check. Then this inner balance can be lost, with negative consequences to our health. (For this reason, beneficial bacteria should always be supplemented following a course of antibiotics.)

Drugs such as penicillin and other forms of antibiotics were developed to combat bacterial infections. The success of these drugs has enabled us to have increased control over many bacterial diseases, including near eradication of many bacterial diseases in industrial nations, such as cholera, leprosy, plague, and typhoid fever. However, more and more bacteria are becoming drug-resistant. It's likely that the simplicity of bacteria allows them to be much more adaptable than other life-forms, evolving strategies that enable them to evade certain antibiotic medications and antibacterial products.

Their simple cell structure also enables them to transfer genetic material to other bacteria, with the ability to quickly pass on antibiotic-resistant traits, even to different species of bacteria. Just such a case has occurred with vancomycin, the antibiotic considered the drug of last resort. Bacterial resistance has developed to vancomycin, and vancomycin-resistant enterococcus bacteria have shared their genetic material with Staphylococcus aureus, enabling the staph bacteria to also become resistant.

The adaptability of bacteria makes it essential that we use multiple strategies in our own defense. Later in this book, you'll find ideas for minimizing your exposure to bacteria.

Strategies for Coexisting with Bacteria

- **Keep your immune system strong.** It's useful to know that more than 60 percent of us carry strep and staph bacteria in our bodies, yet we usually don't develop infection. Under the wrong conditions, these same bacteria can even cause fatal illness. This makes clear the importance of strong immunity to maintain balance within the body—always our first strategy. (See Table 3.3 to read about the effects of stress on beneficial bacteria.)
- **Educate yourself about minimizing exposure.** The most common infectious illnesses worldwide tend to

Table 3.3 Effects of Stress on Beneficial Bacteria

Stressor	How they can be harmful	Potentially harmful microbes
Stress	Can cause changes in composition of the digestive tract lining; beneficial flora may be washed away	*E. coli,* bacteroides, and candida
Diet	High consumption of meat can inhibit beneficial bacteria, with the potential for overgrowth of *E. coli* and clostridium; high consumption of dairy products can encourage strep overgrowth	Too much meat—*E. coli* and clostridium; too many dairy products —strep overgrowth
Antibiotics	Eradicate both harmful and beneficial bacteria; this leaves the digestive tract open to overgrowth by bacteria and yeast in the gut normally considered benign	*Clostridium difficile,* *E. coli*, staph, and strep; yeasts, especially candida

SOURCE: Content provided courtesy of DiagnosTechs, Kent, WA, 1998.

be those spread person-to-person. See Part 2 for more information on cutting your exposure due to:

- Respiratory transmission, which occurs most often in overcrowded environments or when people are indoors in the winter
- Oral-fecal transmission through food handling or touch
- Sexually transmitted diseases
- **Wash your hands often.** Practice good hygiene and housekeeping. The goal is not to eliminate bacteria—this wouldn't be practical or even beneficial. The

strategy is to decrease the level of bacteria in your environment, food and water, and person-to-person exposures to a level your immune system can handle.

- **Promote healthy digestion.** Drink lots of water. Eat a diet of fresh food, low in sugar and simple starches (these are the preferred food of many bacteria). Take friendly flora supplements. Keep your body slightly alkaline by eating at least one salad a day. You can also take other forms of green supplements to maintain the proper acid-alkaline balance.

Our goal is to coexist with the bacteria. They are not about to disappear. Bacteria are believed to be the oldest life-form on earth, dating back 3 billion years. Scientists have also discovered there is no place on earth without bacteria. These microbes have even been found 10,000 feet beneath the surface of the earth, where they survive without oxygen, with pressures up to 3000 pounds per square inch and temperatures up to 185°F.

Viruses

Tim first came to the Health Action Clinic in Santa Barbara as a patient seeking health care and acupuncture to help him cope with HIV. He also participated in a support group for people with chronic illness, which focused on optimizing lifestyle, and he took a Qigong class. When Tim dropped out of sight, the clinic staff assumed they might not see him again. This was in the early years of the AIDS epidemic, and most of the patients with HIV were dying quite young.

The clinic director met Tim again years later, while teaching a Qigong class at a conference in San Francisco. After the class, Tim introduced himself. He was not only surviving HIV—he exuded radiant health. He said that although his job required him to travel, he always made it a point to get involved in a support group and a Qigong class. He felt that these two factors had been instrumental in maintaining his good health.[1]

Overview

The AIDS epidemic has taught us how brilliantly designed and formidable viruses can be. They are among the most mysterious of all microbes. Since their discovery about 100 years ago, researchers have debated whether viruses are living entities or lifeless particles. They are highly streamlined, with no cellular structure or composition. These microbes do not grow, have no metabolism, use no energy, and produce no waste products— and they do not adapt to their environment.

Viruses are capable of reproducing—this is the one quality they share in common with all other life-forms. However, a virus can replicate only after infecting a host cell. In the process of causing infection and reproducing, viruses live harbored inside the host's cells. This is made possible by their minute size— 1 percent of the size of the smallest bacteria. Viruses are so small that an image of a virus produced by an electron microscope must be magnified more than 200,000 times to be at all visible.

Potential Risk

Viruses cause a wide variety of diseases, ranging from the common cold and cold sores to AIDS and cancer. (See Table 3.4 for

Table 3.4   Most Prevalent Viruses Tracked by the CDC

Chicken pox (varicella)	98,727
AIDS	40,758
Hepatitis, all forms	24,630
Life-threatening influenzae	1,398

Source: Data from CDC. Summary of Notifiable Diseases—United States, 2000. *Morbidity and Mortality Weekly Report.* 2002, June 14; 49 (53): 1-102.

a list of the most prevalent viruses in the United States.) Each type of virus is transmitted in a particular way, and some target a specific area of the body. For example, although you can inhale viruses that cause colds and flu, you can't inhale the AIDS virus. In general, the most frequent forms of transmission occur:

- In food and water (such as hepatitis A)
- Through direct contact (HIV)
- By insect bite (West Nile virus)
- Through tiny inhaled water droplets, probably the most common route of viral infection.[2]

The Importance of a Strong Immune Function

We want to remind you again of the importance of maintaining strong immunity in the face of day-to-day exposures to viruses. A textbook description of the importance of immunity states, "Once the host is infected, the host's immune status and competence are probably the major factors that determine whether a viral infection causes a life-threatening disease, a benign lesion, or no symptoms at all."[3] Factors known to affect the severity of a virus include the tissue targeted, the strain of virus, the level of exposure, and the health of the infected person.

When symptoms do develop, it's important to nip them in the bud to conserve immune defenses. For example, flu is known to be one of the types of viral infection that can cause immune suppression. When we can successfully minimize the severity of the flu, we have a better chance of avoiding other secondary infections.

Some viral infections are latent and do not begin to replicate until they are triggered to reproduce. Researchers do not yet fully understand what causes these changes. We do know that in the case of herpes simplex (which causes cold sores), stress or immune suppression can reactivate the virus, resulting in visible symptoms.

How Viruses Work

Viruses can be compared to an incredibly efficient machine with only a few working parts. Viruses consist of either two or three major components:

1. A strand of nucleic acid that contains genetic information—the nucleic acid may be DNA (deoxyribonucleic acid) or RNA (ribonucleic acid), but never both.
2. A layer of protein that encloses these strands, forming a capsule-like structure (a capsid).
3. An additional layer present in certain viruses—an outer envelope of fatty material.

Viruses replicate through any of a variety of complex processes. They may use some of the host's resources, such as genetic material—and may also "hijack" the host's equipment for genetic duplication. Viruses can cause:

- **Acute, immediate infections.** In some infections, the virus produces many new virus particles (for example, polio or flu) and destroys some of the body's cells in the process.
- **Persistent infections.** In other infections, such as hepatitis B, the virus may remain in the cell without destroying it and continue to release new infective viruses at a slower rate. These persistent infections eventually cause the disease to be spread more widely in the population. The infected person may act as a symptomless carrier for a long period of time and remain a continuing source of infection.
- **Latent infections.** In these infections, the virus remains dormant and can be activated by factors such as stress or immune suppression. Chicken pox virus, latent in the body's cells, can reemerge later in life as an inflammation of the nerve cells—shingles. The HIV virus can remain dormant for 1 to 10 years before it manifests as full-blown AIDS.

Many viruses are very specific in the species and organ system they target. For example, the common cold typically affects only the upper respiratory tract. Other viruses such as influenza are very general in their effects and can cause disease in various areas of the body. For example, herpes simplex 2, which causes genital herpes, can be life-threatening to a newborn if the infant is infected as it passes through the birth canal. Like any infectious agent, their effects are a greater threat to those without sufficient immune protection. Table 3.5 shows the ways viruses can be transmitted.

Table 3.5 Virus Transmission

Most frequent means of transmission

Respiratory transmission	Adenoviruses 3, 4, and 7 (which causes respiratory infections, atypical pneumonia), chicken pox, the common cold, fifth disease (parvovirus B19, which causes symptoms that resemble rubella), influenza A and B, measles, mumps, pneumovirus (primary cause of infant lower respiratory tract infections), rubella (German measles), smallpox
Fecal-oral transmission transmission	Coxsackie and echo virus (cause meningitis), hepatitis A and E, Norwalk virus (also found in shellfish, which cause dysentery), rotavirus (primary cause of diarrhea in children)

Other modes of transmission

Animals and insects	Animals: aseptic meningitis (from mice—dangerous to pregnant women), rabies Insects: Colorado tick fever, dengue fever, yellow fever, West Nile virus
Blood	Cytomegalovirus; fifth disease; HIV; human T-cell leukemia/lymphoma; hepatitis B, C, and D
Contact (lesions, saliva, etc.)	Chicken pox, common cold, Epstein-Barr virus (which causes mononucleosis through oral/intimate contact), herpes simplex 1, rabies (through bodily fluids—for example, to health-care workers)
Genetic	Mad cow disease (prions), retroviruses (a class of complex viruses that includes HIV)
Mother to newborn	Chicken pox, cytomegalovirus, echovirus, fifth disease (parvovirus B 19), herpes simplex 2, HIV, human papilloma virus, human T-cell leukemia/lymphoma, rubella (German measles)
Sexual contact	Cytomegalovirus, Epstein-Barr virus (oral/intimate contact; kissing [saliva]), HIV, hepatitis C, herpes simplex 2, human papillomavirus, human T-cell leukemia/lymphoma

SOURCE: Information drawn from Peter Q. Warinner, M.D. *Clinical Microbiology Review*. Long Island, NY: Wysteria, 2001.

Special Issues: Viruses and Cancer

Viruses are now known to play a role in the development of certain cancers. These viruses can "transform" the host cell into a tumor or cancer cell. The cells then "become invasive and can form tumors if injected into animals."[4] These changes come about after viral nucleic acid—viral oncogenes—is incorporated into the host's genetic material. Viruses known to cause cancer include:

- Hepatitis B and C (cancer of the liver)
- Epstein-Barr virus, associated with African Burkitt's lymphoma, Hodgkin's lymphoma, and certain cancers of the nose and throat
- Herpes virus 8, which can result in Kaposi's sarcoma, associated with AIDS
- Human papillomavirus (types 16 and 18), now believed to cause 80 to 90 percent of cervical cancer
- Human adult T-cell leukemia[5]

Minimizing the Impact of Viruses

The following strategies are recommended to hospital personnel and to some extent can be adapted or applied in our own lives.

- **Limiting personal contact with viruses.** This might mean minimizing exposure to crowded public places during the height of flu season, if that is an option. It may also mean rescheduling social engagements when we know that it entails exposure to others who are ill.
- **Being scrupulous about hygiene** (including hand washing!), sanitation, and disinfection.
- **Getting immunized.**

- **Decreasing high-risk behaviors.** For example, take precautions with regard to sexually transmitted diseases.
- **Making sure that the water you drink is as clean as possible.** Purchase bottled water from a supplier that tests for viruses, or use a state-of-the-art filter. (See Chapter 5 for various options.)
- **Becoming skilled in the use of home first aid at the first sign of cold or flu.**
- **Considering using integrative or natural medicine as an option.** For example, when the flu persists, either intravenous vitamin C therapy or acupuncture can be an effective way to speed healing.
- **Maintaining strong immunity.** The immune system's marvelous defenses do not occur by accident. Their vigor is a direct reflection of our own personal health. Research has shown that the ability of defensive immune cells (macrophages), to engulf invaders depends on the availability of certain essential nutrients. Maintaining good nutrition strengthens your immune defenses.

Parasites—Protozoa

A Case of Undetected Infection

When he was about 6, Tony started having problems connected with his digesiton. Tests for parasites came out negative. The doctor said it was ulcerative colitis and put Tony on a variety of medications, including steroids. However,

---

A Case of Undetected Infection (*continued*)

his condition didn't improve; in fact, it grew worse. More tests were performed. An infection caused by amoebas was detected—*Entamoeba histolytica*—a common but aggressive amoeba. Based on the information from the lab test, Tony's doctor prescribed medication targeted at clearing the parasite and his symptoms resolved.

It is impossible to determine if the *E. histolytica* infection caused the ulcerative colitis (which it can do) or if existing inflammation made him more vulnerable to the *E. histolytica*. It is clear that the parasite was a factor in his colitis, because once the parasite was cleared, the ulcerative colitis condition resolved.

Overview

Protozoa are microscopic, single-celled organisms that are parasites in humans and animals. We often think of parasites as occurring only in the tropics, but they also can be found in temperate areas. Many are transmitted through food and water and affect the digestive tract. These species can also be transmitted by those who prepare food in restaurants or in the home. Antiparasitic treatment is often effective against protozoa, but unfortunately, these infections tend to be difficult to identify through laboratory testing. As a result, they frequently go untreated. Protozoa also occur in a wide variety of other forms, such as trichomonas, which can be transmitted sexually, and malaria, which is carried by mosquitoes.

Potential Risk

Worldwide, infectious diarrhea is the second most deadly condition, fatal to 3 million people a year, primarily children, due in part to protozoa and bacteria. The most prevalent kinds of protozoa in temperate climates are shown in Table 3.6

Parasitic infection can damage humans by direct injury to the tissue of the digestive tract, the liver, or other organ systems. In addition, the most destructive effects can be caused by the toxic by-products of parasites. They can disrupt digestive activity, interfere with the action of digestive enzymes, and create nutritional deficiencies. They can also compromise the immune system in order to assure their own survival. These infections can cause chronic fatigue, difficulty with mental concentration, depression, and neurological symptoms. They can also be a factor in conditions such as allergies, asthma, arthritis, food cravings, skin conditions, and other chronic health problems.

Many people who are infected with parasites have no apparent symptoms. Thus they can unknowingly go untreated and pass the condition on to others. As a result, we may be seri-

---

Table 3.6 Estimated Prevalence of Parasitic Infections

Protozoa	Incidence in the United States	Incidence worldwide, estimated
Protozoa affecting the digestive tract		
Amoebas	Most prevalent protozoa in the United States	63 million; 40,000 to 100,000 deaths yearly
Giardia	2 million, estimated	200 million
Cryptosporidium	3128 cases reported	
Protozoa affecting blood and tissue—tropical		
Malaria	1560 reported	400 to 490 million; 2 to 2.5 million deaths
Trypanosomiasis	n.a.	24 million
Leishmaniasis	n.a.	1.2 million

SOURCES: Incidence in the U.S.—data from CDC. Summary of Notifiable Diseases—United States, 2000. *Morbidity and Mortality Weekly Report.* 2002, June 14; 49 (53); 1–102. Estimated worldwide incidence—data from E. K. Markell, D. T. John, and W. A. Krotoski, ed. *Markell and Voge's Medical Parasitology,* 8th ed. Philadelphia: W. B. Saunders, 1999.

ously underestimating parasites as contributors to human disease. Lab testing suggests that parasites are surprisingly common. For example, in one survey of 5792 lab samples, more than one-third (38 percent) of the patients tested positive for parasites.[6] A summary of the types of infections detected from that study are listed in Table 3.7, in order of prevalence. [Note that data on giardiasis is not reported in this particular study.]

Table 3.7   A Review of Parasitic Infection, 2000

Microbe and percentage of those infected	Digestive symptoms reported by patients	General symptoms reported by patients
Amoebas (*Entamoeba histolytica*), 15%	Bloating, flatulence, cramps, diarrhea, constipation	Insomnia, fatigue, nausea, allergies, pain, weight loss
Blastocystis, 8%	Bloating, flatulence, cramps, diarrhea, constipation, poor digestion and poor absorption	Fatigue, nausea, allergies, pain, nervous disorders, skin conditions, muscle problems
Amoebas (*E. coli*), 8%	Bloating, flatulence, cramps, diarrhea, constipaton, irritable bowel syndrome	Fatigue, nausea, allergies, headache depression, lack of concentration, irritability, joint and back pain, skin problems
Amoebas (*E. hartmanni*), 8%	Bloating, flatulence, cramps, irritable bowel syndrome	Nausea, allergies, and pain; disorders of the nervous system, respiratory tract, and skin
Cyclospora, 2%	Symptoms that come and go, bloating, flatulence, cramps, diarrhea	Fatigue, nausea, anemia, headaches, depression, muscle aches, itching

SOURCE: Omar Amin, *A Review of 5,792 Samples*. Phoenix, AZ: Parasitology Center, Inc., 2002.

Where and How Are They Encountered?

In the United States, we consider the problem of parasites an exception—a rarity. We assume we've eradicated parasites with modern sanitation and water treatment. But the data suggest that parasitic infection occurs with surprising frequency and that the incidence is increasing. In many cases, these infections, contracted primarily in food and water, underlie familiar digestive disorders and other conditions as well.

- Cryptosporidium, a waterborne microbe, was reported to cause illness in more than 400,000 people in Milwaukee in 1993. Over 4000 were hospitalized, and at least 100 died.[7] Cryptosporidium is found in the public water systems and reservoirs of many American cities. In some places, such as the San Francisco Bay Area, it is known to be transmitted by the runoff from hillsides where cattle graze, upstream from unprotected reservoirs. Doctors report that all over the United States, these infections occur every day.
- Giardia is often spread as a waterborne infection and is on the rise. In 1997, the Wall Street Journal reported an average of 2 million cases annually in the United States.[8] Worldwide, infection due to giardia is estimated to affect more than 200 million people.[9]
- Cyclospora is an "emerging pathogen" first identified in 1987. In 1996, it caused an outbreak due to contamination of Guatemalan strawberries and raspberries. However, it is also domestic and common in the United States. Like many protozoa, it can be transferred in stool, on human hands, and as contaminates in food and water.

Minimizing Exposure

In this section of the book, you'll find suggestions on cutting your germ exposure in many of the following situations. The greatest risk factors for parasites include:

- Foreign travel (in one study, more than 50 percent of those infected had recently returned from travel)
- Living with a household member who has a parasitic infection (doubles the risk)
- Relapse or reinfection due to a recent parasitic infection

Other factors include:

- Drinking tap water
- Not observing good hygiene
- Dining out often
- Frequenting salad bars
- Being intimate with an infected partner
- Having pets
- Going camping
- Working at an infant-care center
- Living in an institutional setting or group home

Strengthening Your Resistance

Your body has several mechanisms that protect you against digestive parasites. By working with your body, you can strengthen these natural protections:

- Keep your digestive tract operating efficiently by drinking 8 cups of pure water a day and eating enough fiber in fresh fruits, vegetables, and whole grains.

- Listen to your body. Vomiting and diarrhea are the body's mechanical efforts to shed invading microbes. To the degree possible, permit moderate vomiting or diarrhea when it occurs, so your system can perform these vital tasks. Whenever these symptoms are extreme, call your physician.
- Remember that your stomach acid destroys most bad bugs—don't dilute it.
- Don't drink liquid right before, during, or right after a meal.
- Avoid the use of antacid products, including bicarbonate, unless absolutely necessary.
- Use enzymes when needed. Enzymes help digest your food and bad bugs as well. If you have bloating and gas, supplement with enzymes during the meal.
- Take vitamins. Your digestive tract is the site of at least 60 percent of the immunity in your entire body. You can nourish this immunity by taking a good multivitamin and making sure you get enough zinc and vitamin A, available in cod liver oil or other types of vitamin A preparations.

Special Issues: Difficulties in Diagnosis

Detecting and treating parasitic infections can be a complex process. For example, some microorganisms are classified as commensals—they are present but don't actually cause disease. Parasites and bacteria thought to be harmless until recently include certain amoebas, giardia, H. pylori (which causes ulcers), and blastocystis. In the past 10 years, they have been reclassified, because we now know that these organisms and many others can cause serious infections. In fact, some can contribute to illnesses that can linger for years if untreated. Once the infection is found and treated, patients often improve quite rapidly.

Mold

Ed was sickened by toxic mold that spread through his home when a pipe burst, flooding the den with water. Mold was found in the den a month later and had spread to other parts of the house, including the air conditioning ducts. Ed and his wife both became seriously ill. He developed a severe cough and congestion that lasted for months, requiring that he take antibiotics and cancel several speaking engagements. Their dog died from illness that was mold-related. At that point, the couple moved out of their multimillion dollar home into a rental house so that repairs could be performed. However, months later, the removal of the toxic mold still had not been completed. This is a true story, and unfortunately occurs all too often due to the extreme difficulty of removing mold in building structures.[10]

Overview

We're hearing more in the media about the toxic effects of mold. Why? Molds are becoming more widely recognized as a cause of human illness. They are not contagious like bacteria and viruses—they're not transmitted from one person to another. Molds are not usually a direct cause of infectious illness, although they do seem to be a contributing factor. More often, they trigger symptoms of allergies or sensitivities. Responses can range from mild, temporary reactions to acute or chronic illness. The symptoms can occur as a result of exposure to mold spores, mold toxins, or their by-products and may include:

- Nasal or sinus congestion
- Flu-like symptoms or cough
- Bronchitis, asthma, or pneumonia
- Lack of concentration or memory impairment
- Dizziness, headaches, or nausea
- Skin rashes or irritation
- Weakened immunity

People with inherited allergies are much more likely to also develop allergic reactions to molds, once they are exposed to a particular mold and become sensitized to it. Since about 1 in 10 Americans suffers from allergy-related sinus conditions or asthma, the number of people who are actually affected by mold may be extensive. Estimates range as high as 25 million people.

What Are Molds?

Molds, yeast, and mushrooms are all types of fungus. Molds are among the most widespread of all living organisms, with tens of thousands of different varieties. Unlike plants, they cannot produce their own nourishment, rather, they gain sustenance by breaking down organic matter. Many molds have a base of hair-fine, root-like appendages that enable them to anchor and absorb nutrients. The upper portion of these complex, multicellular structures is composed of branching thread-like filaments. Many species of mold reproduce through seed-like spores, which are produced in the filaments and released into the air. In addition, molds produce volatile organic compounds—waste products given off as they decompose the material in their environment.

Mold colonies are highly active, in contrast to yeasts, which consist of single passive cells. For example, one 4-inch spot of mold can produce millions of spores. The spores may give off toxins, termed mycotoxins, which are capable of producing allergic-type sensitivity. They also can suppress the immune system. Exposure to a mold colony this size can be enough to trigger an asthma attack.

Potential Risk

There have been more than a thousand studies on the effects of mold. Three studies of general interest found a correlation between the presence of mold and illness.

- The Mayo Clinic tested 210 patients with chronic sinus conditions. Researchers found that 96 percent of the patients had fungus in their mucus.[11]
- Another study, conducted in Finland, involved surveying more than 10,000 university students. The survey inquired about the dampness of their homes, whether they had asthma or other allergies, and how often they developed colds and other respiratory infections. Students who reported visible mold in their homes were more than twice as likely to have asthma.[12]
- A study conducted in the Netherlands evaluated 259 children with chronic respiratory symptoms and compared their medical histories with 257 children who had no symptoms. Among the children with respiratory symptoms, testing found that 24 children had elevated antibodies to mold. (Antibodies are an immune defense. This study tested for antibodies specific to mold, which would suggest the presence of a mold allergy.) Among the children with no symptoms, only 2 had elevated mold antibodies. The

study also concluded that there was a connection between damp conditions in the home and sensitization to molds.[13]

The study of mold as an environmental toxin is a growing field that is beginning to have an impact on medicine, law, real estate, and public policy. At the time of this writing, legal standards have not been set that would define what constitutes a mold hazard. Federal standards have been legislated for certain industrial toxins, but the safe level of mold exposure has not yet been specified. Consequently, homeowners and tenants have no legal recourse when their home or health is destroyed by toxic mold.

One of the molds of greatest concern is stachybotrys, or black mold. This particular fungus can cause bleeding in the lungs, which can be potentially fatal for infants and pregnant women. When stachybotrys spores are inhaled into the lungs, they can weaken blood vessels and may cause nosebleeds or bleeding elsewhere in the body. This mold is found in wet areas (for example, where there is a leak in the home) and is black and slimy and smears when touched.

Where and When Molds Occur

Mold can grow any time and any place, as long as there is moisture and a source of nourishment. It thrives in warmth and high humidity, so summer seasons and humid climates favor the growth of mold. Within the home, mold can grow year-round in showers and refrigerators. Since it flourishes in dark, damp, poorly ventilated areas, basements and crawl spaces are natural mold habitats. If you have symptoms of mold allergy, it's important to carefully evaluate your home or have it evaluated. It is essential to identify any possible water leakage within the walls or the structure, poor drainage that may cause excessive dampness in the basement or foundation, areas of standing water, or other areas that can harbor dampness. Common sources of indoor moisture that may lead to mold problems include:

- Leaky roofs, plumbing leaks, and overflow from sinks or drains
- A damp basement or crawl space under the house
- Steam from the shower, from cooking, or steam from a humidifier
- A dryer exhaust that is vented indoors
- Flooding

Mold that grows outside can become widely dispersed through the air and enter the home through the windows. An air conditioner with a good filter is one strategy for stopping the flow of exterior mold into your home if you are highly sensitive or if you live in a situation that increases your exposure. Drainage problems near the house need to be corrected since pooled water greatly increases mold formation. Mold can congregate in the soil, leaf or compost piles, sandboxes, garages, and barns. People with asthma or sensitivity also want to remember that natural settings such as the forest harbor mold as part of the ecosystem of decaying logs and vegetation.

One of the challenges that airborne molds present is that they are difficult to discern or detect. Related health problems can be difficult to clearly identify and diagnose. Mold exposures may be subtle if the mold is not visible and there is no musty scent. You may not even realize that molds are affecting your health because they can be ever-present in the environment. These chronic exposures often occur over a period of months or years.

It is important not to live, work, or stay for long periods of time in a place that smells of mildew or mold, or that you know harbors mold. Although you may have done all you can to clear mold residues that are visible, there can also be mold growth under the carpet, in overstuffed furniture or cushions, or clinging to books or papers. In the worst cases, mold can invade the duct system of the house, or wooden or concrete structures, continuing to produce hazardous spores or toxins.

Health Problems Due to Molds

Medical research has documented a number of health effects that can result from mold exposure.

- **Airborne molds that cause allergies.** Extensive literature has documented the link between airborne molds and symptoms of allergies or sensitivities.
- **Conditions of the skin and nails.** There are a number of conditions in which fungus grows on the surfaces of the body, on the nails or skin (for example, athlete's foot and ringworm). These conditions tend to be spread by direct contact.
- **Invasive "infections."** Termed deep mycoses, these fungal infections occur mainly in immune-compromised individuals and tend to involve the internal organs.

New perspectives on mold also suggest the potential for other types of health problems.

- **Localized sinus infection.** It is now believed that there are airborne molds that tend to colonize the sinuses and possibly other areas of the respiratory tract. Although this is a fairly new perspective, we do know, as noted earlier, that the Mayo Clinic study on sinusitis found microscopic evidence of mold in the mucus of 96 percent of sinus patients tested.

- **Low-grade mold/fungal hypersensitivity.** We also know that there can be molds in the foods we eat. Some are used for culinary purposes—beer and wine, bread, cheeses, mushroom (a type of fungus), and soy sauce are just a few examples. Other molds are unintentional contaminants in food. We, and numerous other physicians in integrative medicine, have been working with mold-related health issues for more than a decade. An integrative approach involves lab testing to evaluate the possible presence of yeast, such as candida, and treatment using antifungal medication, supplements, and diet. Our observations consistently suggest that molds can have an effect on digestive function, and that people with candida overgrowths in the digestive tract tend to be more sensitive to molds in their food. These conditions also tend to be made worse by a diet high in sugars and starches.
- **Conditions such as chronic fatigue, due to environmental exposure.** We, and other physicians who practice environmental medicine, have found that patients experiencing frequent mold exposure tend to develop respiratory conditions, chronic fatigue, and difficulty with mental tasks. These symptoms are well documented in the medical literature, particularly from the field of occupational medicine.

Minimizing Exposure

Environmental molds can cause problems serious enough to warrant your attention. In fact, the impact of molds on health has not yet been fully appreciated. A brief summary of strategies against environmental mold includes these steps:

- **Remove the source of exposure to the degree possible.** In some situations, basic cleanup and disinfection are sufficient. This may also mean simplifying your home environment and removing carpets, cushions, and other objects that retain mold. (See Chapter 6 for information on cleaning and disinfecting your home.) If you have allergies or sensitivities, you will want either to have someone else do the cleanup or to wear a quality face mask and protective clothing. Be sure to shower and wash your clothes thoroughly afterward.
- **Control moisture.** This is one of the most effective ways to inhibit indoor mold growth. A dehumidifier and a barometer will enable you to maintain the humidity at 35 to 45 percent—it is difficult for mold to grow in an environment with low humidity.
- **Consider the use of an air purifier.** A number of excellent brands are on the market. You'll want to do careful research before purchasing one.
- **Consider medical treatment.** You may want to seek testing and treatment by an integrative physician who specializes in this area, if your problems seem mold-related and persist after the exposure is removed.
- **Move to another building (*or to a drier climate*).** Some people have found it necessary to relocate in

order to restore their health. Additional strategies for eradication are listed in Chapter 7 on airborne transmission.

Insect-Borne Diseases

Jason was in his second year of college when he became ill, following a camping trip. His doctor assumed it was a case of flu and followed his progress. However, Jason did not recover and was unable to resume his studies. He grew worse and eventually suffered the loss of his vision. After much searching, his family located our practice because of our experience in the diagnosis and treatment of Lyme disease. Although we were able to treat Jason for the Lyme disease, it was too late to restore his sight.

Overview

Microbes that cause disease can be transmitted through a variety of insects. The diseases most familiar in the United States are Lyme disease, transmitted by ticks, and West Nile virus, transmitted by mosquitoes. Worldwide, one of the most prevalent conditions is malaria, also transmitted by mosquitoes.

Potential Risk, Location, and Season

The risk of insect-transmitted infectious illness is increasing. In the United States, Lyme disease is the most prevalent of these, with almost 18,000 cases reported in the year 2000.[14] Since Lyme disease resembles a number of other infectious conditions and is extremely difficult to diagnose, it is likely that its occurrence is vastly underreported. The potential for transmission is increasing as well. In New York State, for example, an estimated 60 percent of all ticks carry Lyme. Rocky Mountain spotted fever is another tick-borne illness caused by the bacteria rickettsia. This disease is rarer in the East than Lyme disease, with the highest potential for transmission in the Colorado area.

The West Nile virus continues to spread across the United States, with 1400 reported cases by the end of summer 2002 and 64 confirmed deaths. The CDC reports that the potential for infection currently remains extremely low—1 percent chance of being bitten by an infected mosquito, and of those bitten, 1 percent chance of developing the virus.

Transmission

Transmission of all these illnesses occurs through an insect bite. In the case of Lyme, a rash and/or flu-like symptoms may occur. Since the primary seasons for transmission are summer and fall, any illness with flu-like symptoms at that time of year should be considered suspect and checked with a physician knowledgeable in the treatment of these conditions. With the West Nile virus, no symptoms occur at the time of transmission, but since it affects the brain and nervous system, any flu-like illness that causes headaches, mental confusion, or delirium should be evaluated immediately by a physician.

Prevention

Preventive measures include protective efforts when in a natural or wooded environment.

- Using insect repellent, wearing long pants tucked into one's socks, and wearing long-sleeve shirts
- Checking frequently for ticks

- Limiting outdoor activity at dawn, dusk, and early evening when insects are most active
- Reducing mosquito breeding grounds whenever possible by draining birdbaths, fountains, and other sources of standing water
- Spraying insecticides to limit the population of mosquitoes

Treatment

Treatment options for Lyme disease include the extended use of antibiotics to fully erradicate the infection. Supportive therapy with nutrition is also helpful. West Nile virus currently has no treatment other than interventions that support the immune function.

Prions—Mad Cow Disease

Overview

Prions have been described as "unconventional slow viruses."[15] Like viruses, they are too small to be visible except under a very powerful microscope, and they can transmit disease. Otherwise, they do not conform to the classic profile of a virus. Prions are bits of protein that cause diseases of the central nervous system—diseases that can resemble dementia, Alzheimer's disease, or multiple sclerosis, characterized by trembling and loss of mental function. Prion diseases in humans include kuru (once evident in cannibalistic populations in New Guinea) and Creutzfeldt-Jakob disease. In animals, prions cause scrapie (in sheep and goats) and mad cow disease (bovine spongiform encephalopathy—BSE). In the past 10 years, the most prevalent form of prion disease has been mad cow disease, which occurred in a series of outbreaks in Great Britain.

Potential Risk, Location, and Season

Strong evidence has accumulated for a causal relationship between European outbreaks of mad cow disease (BSE) and a disease in humans called Creutzfeldt-Jakob disease (CJD). Both disorders are ultimately fatal brain diseases with unusually long incubation periods, conditions which take years to develop. According to the CDC, as of July 2002, cattle remain the only known food animal species with disease caused by the BSE agent. During the epidemic in Great Britain, more than 178,000 cases of BSE in cattle were reported (from 1986 to 1999).[16] At least 98 percent of cases of BSE worldwide were reported from the United Kingdom, where the disease was first described.[17] By 2001, 18 other nations had reported at least one case of BSE.

A total of 124 human cases of CJD were reported in the United Kingdom, six cases in France, and one case each in Ireland, Italy, and the United States, from 1995 through June 2002. The patients from Ireland and the United States had each lived in the United Kingdom for more than 5 years during the BSE epidemic in the United Kingdom. There appears to be no seasonal pattern to the transmission.

Transmission

In some cases the condition is inherited, but, in general, transmission of prions occurs through infected tissue. Currently, the primary risk occurs in medical settings, to surgeons and to transplant and brain surgery patients. There is also some risk to people who receive electroencephalograms, so it is important that electrodes and neurosurgical tools be disinfected according to recommendations.

Although some researchers feel there is not sufficient proof to link mad cow disease to consumption of beef cattle, during the epidemic in Britain the number of cases declined significantly once cattle were no longer fed meat byproducts— a drop in the number of cases by more than 60 percent over a 3-year period.

The current risk of acquiring CJD from eating beef and beef products in the United Kingdom appears to be extremely small, perhaps about one case per 10 billion servings. In other countries of the world, the current risk, if it exists at all, would not likely be any higher than that in the United Kingdom. Milk and milk products from cows are not believed to pose any risk for transmitting the BSE agent. To reduce the possible current risk of acquiring CJD from food, travelers to Europe or other areas with increased risk or with known cases of BSE may wish to consider:

1. Avoiding beef and beef products altogether
2. Selecting beef or beef products, such as solid pieces of muscle meat (rather than calf brains or mixed beef products such as burgers and sausages)

Prevention

Mad cow disease is difficult to diagnose, and currently no tests are available. Once the disease is fully present, MRI findings show certain characteristic patterns in the brain. Prion-related diseases can cause progressive loss of memory, cognitive ability, and speech, as well as blindness and symptoms of mental ill-ness. As a result, these conditions are often mistaken for other neurological disorders and types of dementia. The incubation period is 1 to 30 years, but once symptoms are evident, the aver-age life span is less than 8 months.

Treatment

There is currently no known form of treatment. Fortunately, the incidence has dropped to very low levels since 1998, with a total worldwide of fewer than 6000 cases of BSE.

Large Parasites—the Helminths

Overview

Among the various parasites, most helminths are not micro-scopic, nor are they considered microbes. Helminths cause bil-lions of infections each year. Consequently, their role in human disease is so important that we mention them here. There are three primary classifications of helminths: roundworms (nema-todes), flukes (trematodes), and tapeworms (cestodes).

Nematodes of medical importance include hookworm, pinworm, roundworm (ascaris), and whipworm. Pinworm is the most common helminthic infection in North America, and occurs in crowded conditions such as day-care centers, schools, and other institutional settings. Roundworm (ascaris) is the most common worldwide, with an estimated 1.3 billion people infected.[18] Cestodes are various types of tapeworms; many affect humans and are transmitted by animals. Trema-todes are flukes of various types, including liver and lung flukes, as well as blood flukes (schistosoma). Once associated only with tropical regions, schistosoma is now found in some U.S. lakes, causing a condition called swimmer's itch.

Transmission

Various helminths can be transmitted if sanitation is poor through contaminated water and food and through transmission by food handlers. Helminths can also be conveyed by pets such as cats and dogs, by farm animals such as swine, and through contact with soil or sandboxes that contain animal feces. Crowded settings and close contact can promote transmission in schools, institutional settings, and in the home. Protozoa and various types of helminths can also be sexually transmitted.

Prevention

Preventive measures include good personal hygiene, clipping of fingernails and use of a fingernail brush, thorough washing of bed clothes, and prompt treatment of all infected individuals in the household. When housecleaning is performed in the home of an infected family, dusting should be done with a damp mop.

Treatment

In these cases, antihelminthic medications are the choice of treatment, and all members in a household should be treated at one time to avoid reintroduction of the organism and reinfection. Although cure rates are high, reinfection is common. A second course of treatment after 2 weeks can be useful in preventing reinfection.

Toxic Algae

Overview

Health problems associated with toxic algae have been increasing over the past decade. "Toxic species constitute a very small percentage of the thousands of species of microscopic algae at the base of the marine food chain. However, when these species proliferate, they may cause massive kills of fish and shellfish, the death of marine mammals and seabirds, alterations in marine habitats, and with . . . exposure, human illness and death."[19]

When the levels of toxic algae increase, sea life is affected. People who eat or handle toxic seafood can develop symptoms. Exposure can also occur by breathing water vapor containing the algae or through skin contact. Health conditions associated with toxic algae include:

- Amnesic shellfish poisoning
- Ciguatera fish poisoning
- Diarrhetic shellfish poisoning
- Neurotoxic shellfish poisoning
- Paralytic shellfish poisoning
- Pfiesteria-associated syndrome

Location

Harmful algae blooms appear to be increasing in frequency and have been identified at a growing number of sites worldwide. Some are concentrated in continental U.S., Canadian, or Alaskan coastal waters. Other toxic blooms have caused shellfish poisoning near France, Spain, and other parts of Europe, as well as Japan, the South Pacific, and the Caribbean. Although increased incidence of toxic algal blooms are not well understood, they may be related to climate change and disruption of ecosystems. In the United States, particularly in North Carolina and the Chesapeake Bay waters, toxic exposure due to pfiesteria has been linked to nutrient enrichment of waterways from runoff of poultry and hog farms.

Potential Risk

Human illness due to biotoxins from toxic algae is caused by ingesting fish or seafood that has consumed the toxic algae, breathing the spray from ocean waves that contain the algae, or in some cases, having direct skin contact with water containing the toxins. The three primary types of symptoms are gastrointestinal symptoms, neurological symptoms, and localized irritation to the eyes, respiratory tract, or skin. Neurological symptoms follow unusual patterns. In some cases, they can be life threatening, as with amnesic or paralytic shellfish poisoning, found in the United States and Canada. In other cases, the symptoms are temporary, for example in cases of ciguatera fish poisoning, which is the most common marine biotoxin poisoning worldwide. The syndrome associated with pfiesteria is also temporary, and although it causes severe learning deficits, the symptoms are completely reversed once exposure ceases. (See Table 3.8 for a summary of the effects caused by shellfish poisoning related to algae blooms.)

Prevention

The most effective form of prevention is to avoid exposure. This means being aware of the sources of shellfish and other fish you

Table 3.8 Shellfish Poisoning Linked to Toxic Algae

Type of illness	Source of exposure	Gastrointestinal and other symptoms	Neurological symptoms
Amnesic shellfish poisoning	Eating toxic shellfish such as clams—Altantic coast of Canada; Monterey Bay, CA	Gastroenteritis: vomiting, abdominal cramps, diarrhea	Headache; memory loss—severe if exposure is intense with long-term symptoms
Ciguatera fish poisoning—most common marine biotoxin worldwide	Eating toxic barracuda or jack fish—occurs across the globe, and in Caribbean and South Pacific reefs	Acute gastroenteritis	Neurological symptoms lasting weeks to months
Diarrhetic shellfish poisoning	Eating toxic mussels, scallops, or clams—France, Spain, other parts of Europe, Nova Scotia, Japan	Acute gastroenteritis: diarrhea, nausea, vomiting, or abdominal pain	
Neurotoxic shellfish poisoning	Eating toxic shellfish or breathing ocean spray—Florida's Atlantic coast	Gastrointestinal symptoms; toxic ocean spray can cause respiratory irritation, asthma-like symptoms	Neurological symptoms
Paralytic shellfish poisoning—most common marine bio-toxin in the United States	Eating toxic clams and mussels—continental United States and Alaska		Acute neurologial symptoms; may cause respiratory paralysis

Table 3.8 *(continued)*

Type of illness	Source of exposure	Gastrointestinal and other symptoms	Neurological symptoms
Pfiesteria-associated syndrome	Breathing spray or having skin contact with water—certain North Carolina rivers, Chesapeake Bay	Acute respiratory and eye irritation	Severe deficiencies in learning and memory, with total recovery once exposure ceases

Source: Information based on Gerald L. Mandell, John E. Bennett, and Raphael Dolin. Chapter 275: Human illness associated with harmful algal blooms. In *Mandell, Douglas, and Bennett's Principles and Practice of Infectious Diseases*, 5th Ed. St. Louis, MO: Churchill Livingston, 2000.

eat. In some areas, public health authorities monitor the levels of toxic algae in waters where shellfish are harvested. Two forms of these biotoxins are associated with breathing waterborne aerosols. Pfiesteria can result from extended exposure to toxins in the water, so those who come in contact with Maryland–Virginia–North Carolina waterways during an active fish kill are encouraged to wear protective clothing and respiratory gear. Another biotoxin, neurotoxic shellfish poisoning, is associated with the red tides that result from algal blooms along the Atlantic coast of Florida. Airborne toxins from ocean spray can also cause respiratory irritation and asthma-like symptoms in people walking along the beaches in the area of a red tide.

2

Minimizing
Your Exposure

4

Food Prep and Kitchen Tips

For many of us, mealtime is an important ritual, while food preparation and cleanup are often considered mundane and tedious tasks. Yet being lax in these important chores can pose risks to our health. Consider your efforts in the kitchen a meaningful contribution to your family's good health.

Our Changing World

When it comes to kitchen hygiene, most of us are aware of the basics—maintaining clean countertops, cupboards, and appliances; cooking foods to temperatures that assure safety; refrigerating perishables whenever they're not in use; and washing our hands before handling food. What may not be so obvious is the important link between hygiene and health.

We know from the news that some of our meat supply contains antibiotic-resistant bacteria and that millions of eggs are contaminated with salmonella. Foods previously thought to be safe, such as orange juice and alfalfa sprouts, may contain deadly bacteria or parasites. It is essential that we adapt our lifestyle and habits to this changing microbial exposure. The best way to cope with illnesses caused by germs is to prevent them. Isn't it better to avoid these problems by washing and cooking them away?

Why are microbes in our food supply an increasing health hazard? One-fourth of our food supply comes from overseas and outside our borders. In fact, in certain seasons, up to 70 percent of the fruits and vegetables consumed in the United States come from Mexico and South America. When we import food, we bring an entire microbial population with it. Our food is also processed on a massive scale, in batches of millions of pounds that are often shipped thousands of miles. The opportunities for contamination have increased astronomically. Foods are often mixed and batched in packing, processing, or serving, mixing contaminated products with those that are clean. This has resulted, for example, in a number of *E. coli* outbreaks and the recall of millions of pounds of beef. In the global market, ingredients from many countries may be combined in a single dish, which makes contamination difficult to track. Microbes are highly adaptable and respond to these opportunities. Simple transgressions in the kitchen can also make the food unsafe. Since some produce and products have a short shelf life, they may be gone before an outbreak is recognized.

From 1973 to 1987, tainted produce accounted for just 2 percent of food-borne illness. From 1988 through 1991, it caused 5 percent of the outbreaks. Now these problems are on the rise—affecting foods from apple juice and cider to lettuce and tomatoes. The safety of our food supply has become a major public health issue.

How Big Is the Problem?

Only about 100,000 cases of food poisoning are reported to the CDC each year, but obviously a lot more cases actually occur. The occurrence is at least 10 times the reported numbers, and projections from the Council for Agricultural Science and Technology are as high as 33 million cases each year. Other estimates range as high as 80 million cases annually.

Food contamination means that a food contains levels of microbes that create a potential risk to human health. This can happen during growing, processing, or shipping, or it can occur due to improper refrigeration—which is the number-one source of contamination. Meats, for example, may be infected even before the animals are slaughtered. Food poisoning can result, primarily caused by bacteria or microscopic parasites. It is estimated that about 9000 people die each year from food-related contamination, about 25 a day. However, only about 1000 cases a year are documented. Taking extra precautions when we prepare food at home helps to minimize contamination by microbes such as bacteria, viruses, protozoa, or molds. The FDA points out that some people are more at risk than others, and for these people both the choice and preparation of foods require greater care. Those most at risk of food poisoning include:

- Children and infants[1]
- Pregnant women
- Older adults
- People with weakened immune systems, such as those with HIV or AIDS or with cancer, leukemia, diabetes, or kidney disease

- People taking steroids or medications for organ transplants
- People on acid blockers, because these medications decrease stomach acid, which is our primary natural protection against microbes

Bacteria That Cause Food Poisoning

A study of traceable cases of food poisoning has found that more than half were caused by contaminated poultry and seafood—about 20 percent chicken and 40 percent fish (mainly shellfish). Only about 10 percent involved viruses. Salmonella, shigella, and campylobacter are the most common bacteria that cause food poisoning (see Table 4.1). They infect animals and are passed on to humans in our food. Other less common illnesses are important because although rare, they can be fatal. These include botulism, listeria, and toxigenic *E coli*. Botulism, the result of a toxin released by the bacteria *Clostridium botulinum*, is not really very common, but it can be fatal. All these bacterial infections usually require medical treatment with antibiotics.

Table 4.1 Causes of Food Poisoning, 1995

Microbe	Source	Reported cases	Estimated cases
Bacteria			
Salmonella	Undercooked poultry, beef, fish; uncooked eggs in eggnog, desserts, etc.; undercooked omelets, quiches, etc.; unpasteurized juices; sprouts	45,970	600,000 to 2,000,000+

Table 4.1 (continued)

Microbe	Source	Reported cases	Estimated cases
		Reported cases	
Bacteria, continued			
Campylobacter	Undercooked poultry, especially giblets and chicken livers; raw milk	10,000+	2,000,000+
Shigella	Transmission by food handlers; potato, tuna, and shrimp salad; poultry; milk and dairy products; raw vegetables	32,080	300,000
E. coli	Meat, raw milk; unpasteurized fruit juices; alfalfa sprouts	2,139	20,000
Listeria	Undercooked beef, poultry; water; unpasteurized soft cheeses; raw milk	1,600* (415 fatal)	1,850+
Botulism	Spoiled home-canned food; spores in honey; contaminated fish	97	Not available (n.a.)
Vibrio (cholera)	Shellfish—oysters and clams	23	n.a.
Yersinia	Undercooked pork, oysters, fish; raw milk	n.a.	17,000
Microscopic parasites			
Cryptosporidium	Drinking water; fruits or juices; sometimes raw vegetables	n.a.	5,000,000+
Amoebas (*E. histolytica*)	Food handlers; sexual contact; drinking water; certain foods	3,328	2,000,000+
Giardia	Drinking water	n.a.	2,000,000
Trichina	Undercooked pork	2	n.a.
Cyclospora	Contaminated water; fruit	n.a.	Rare but debilitating

Table 4.1 *(continued)*

Microbe	Source	Reported cases	Estimated cases
Viruses			
Hepatits A virus	Food handlers; contaminated water, shellfish, or salads	31,582	n.a.
Norwalk virus	Shellfish such as oysters and clams	Unknown	Frequent
Natural toxins			
Mushroom toxins	Specific toxic species of mushrooms	44 cases in 5 years	Rare but can be fatal
Aflatoxins	Peanuts and other nuts; corn, cottonseed, milk	Unknown	n.a.
Ciguatera toxin	Large finfish—jack, mackerel, large grouper, and snapper	Unknown	n.a.
Shellfish toxins	Potentially any shellfish—mussels, clams, oysters, scallops	Unknown	Rare but can be fatal

Sᴏᴜʀᴄᴇs: Reported cases in 1995 from CDC, *Morbidity and Mortality Weekly Report.*. Web site:www.cdc.gov/mmwr/. Additional data from the Food and Drug Administration. Web site: www.cfsan.fda.gov/~dms/unwelcom.html.

Salmonella infection most often comes from contaminated animal protein that has not been fully cooked—rare meats, raw milk and unpasteurized cheeses, and undercooked eggs, poultry, and fish. There are an estimated 2 to 3 million cases of undiagnosed salmonella food poisoning in the United States each year. Salmonella infections cause fever, chills, diarrhea, abdominal pain, sometimes vomiting, and often a severe headache. Fortunately, it is rarely fatal, and these infections respond to treatment with an antibiotic such as ampicillin.

Symptoms usually clear in 1 to 2 days. It has been suggested that the increased bacterial levels in meat are due in some degree to lack of hygiene in some factory farming environments. This is a good reason to moderate the intake of animal protein and to buy organic whenever possible. *In general, salmonella can best be avoided by thoroughly cooking all dishes that include meat, poultry, seafood, or eggs and by using only pasteurized milks and cheeses.*

Campylobacter is another bacterial illness originating in poultry. It can cause diarrhea, cramping, pain, and fever about 2 to 5 days after exposure. Over 10,000 cases are reported to the CDC each year, which estimates that the illness actually affects as many as 2 million persons each year, about 1 percent of the population. Campylobacter occurs more frequently in the summer, and more often to infants and young adults. It is fatal in about 500 cases a year. Poultry is typically the source of campylobacter in 99 percent of cases. *Since poultry can carry campylobacter without becoming ill, the best way to avoid this infection is to cook all poultry thoroughly.*

Infrequent but Serious Causes of Food Poisoning

Shigella is a group of bacteria that also cause gastrointestinal illness, with symptoms of fever, abdominal pain, and diarrhea. The bacteria are transmitted through direct contact, from food handled by someone with an infection, and through contaminated water. Shigella bacteria are most commonly transmitted in milk and dairy products, poultry, tuna, shrimp, and raw vegetables. In 1995, more than 32,000 cases of shigellosis were reported to the CDC, almost double the number 10 years earlier. It can be fatal in about 10 percent of cases. Children and food handlers are most frequently the carriers. *The single most important way to prevent shigellosis is hand washing with soap and running water.*

E. coli is another bacterial illness. A nonharmful form of *E. coli* bacteria occurs naturally in the human digestive tract, but there are four dangerous forms of this microbe. Of these, the strain identified as O157:H7 makes the headlines because of its potential for serious damage to health or even death. Although only about 2000 cases were reported in 1995, it is estimated that more than 20,000 cases of this infection occur in the United States each year. Problems may be severe, including bloody diarrhea and occasionally kidney failure. The primary cause has been undercooked beef, but *E. coli* also is found in raw milk, unpasteurized fruit juices, and sewage-contaminated water. *E. coli* can be transmitted through person-to-person contact in families and in child-care centers. *Since most cases of E. coli have been associated with eating undercooked ground beef, the primary prevention includes cooking beef and hamburgers to at least 160°F on the meat thermometer.*

Listeria is a bacterial infection that is fairly rare, but it can be quite serious. Listeria can cause meningitis, a serious illness that can result in brain injury or death. Although only an estimated 2000 cases of listeria occur each year, 425 of these are fatal—more than 20 percent. Listeria primarily affects those most vulnerable, particularly people with AIDS and pregnant women, and it typically begins with flu-like symptoms. These bacteria are found in soil and water and as a contaminant in manure. Listeria is contracted from raw foods and is found in raw or uncooked meats, hot dogs, poultry, and fish; occasionally raw vegetables or ice cream; in raw milk and unpasteurized cheeses (Camembert, Brie, or Mexican-style cheese); and in contaminated processed foods such as deli cold cuts. *The best way to prevent this life-threatening infection is to avoid foods that are raw or undercooked, such as runny cheeses and rare meats.*

Botulism is a rare but serious food-borne disease, caused by the contamination of food from *Clostridium botulinum* bacteria. Botulism toxins are most frequently transmitted in spoiled home-canned food and occasionally in contaminated fish and other commercial food products. Botulism in infants can be caused by eating the spores of botulinum bacteria, in sources such as honey. Although there are only about 100 cases a year in the United States, botulism can be fatal. *The FDA recommends that children less than a year old not be fed honey and that careful precautions be taken in home canning and the use of home-canned foods. The toxin is destroyed by boiling for 10 minutes, so home-canned food is safest if boiled.*

Other Causes of Food-borne Infection

Hepatitis A can be conveyed through contaminated food or can be contracted from other people, who serve as carriers. Most often, germs are transmitted by those working in fields and factories helping to process food or by those who prepare foods at home or in restaurants. Both shellfish and strawberries have been found to be contaminated with the hepatitis virus. *Most intestinal viruses and bacteria are typically transferred from the hands, so hand washing is an essential protective habit.*

Amoebas are one of the most common parasitic problems worldwide, transmitted in food and water. They can cause a range of symptoms, from mild or periodic indigestion to acute dysentery with fever, chills, and pain. People who handle or prepare food can pass disease-causing amoebas to others. Washing

hands and scrubbing fingernails with a nailbrush before handling food are important steps in preventing the transmission
of amoebas.

Molds are the most common microbes that contaminate
foods. They can grow on cheeses, breads, meats, herbs, nuts,
and grains. In general, most molds are fairly well tolerated
when consumed in small amounts. Some people, however, are
allergic or sensitive to molds. Also, certain molds on foods may
produce specific toxins that can cause serious illness. Aflatox-
ins, produced by the molds *Aspergillus flavus* and *parasiticus*,
are potentially harmful, especially to the liver, where they can
cause a type of hepatitis or even cancer. Mold has been associated most commonly with peanuts but can also contaminate
other nuts and also grains such as corn, wheat, and barley.
Bread and cheese molds may cause allergic-type reactions or
sensitivities, but are generally less harmful. To prevent mold,
buy your food fresh, store or refrigerate it immediately, and
freeze it if you will not be using it within a few days.

Coping with Food Poisoning

How do you know if you have food poisoning? One answer is,
you'll know! The most typical symptoms are diarrhea (the
body's attempt to shed the offending organisms), cramping,
and fever, as well as headache, vomiting, and exhaustion.
Symptoms may develop as quickly as 30 minutes after eating or
may take days or weeks to develop (with listeria, for example).
Food poisoning can last for 24 hours or for a week to 10 days.
When to see the doctor? When the fever is above 102°F or
there is blood or pus in the stool, prolonged vomiting and/or
diarrhea, or dehydration, call the doctor or emergency room
immediately.

Cause for Hope

Given all the concerns, it's helpful to know that our society has coped successfully with such problems in the past. Typhoid fever, which was very common at the beginning of the twentieth century, is now almost forgotten in the United States. It was conquered in the pre-antibiotic era through the treatment of water and sewage, the pasteurization of milk, and improved shellfish sanitation. Similarly, cholera, bovine tuberculosis, and trichinosis have also been successfully controlled in this country. Today, in what some are calling the post-antibiotic era, it is essential that we return to good hygiene and other preventive approaches to avoid illness.

Situation (Location): Selecting and Purchasing Food

Fact

The total number of reported food poisoning cases in 1995 — more than 100,000
Estimated cases in 2002 — more than 76 million annually

Sources of Exposure

Food workers and handlers; inadequate refrigeration

Germs and Risk

Salmonella and campylobacter, each estimated to affect more than 2 million people yearly

Overview

Although you can't control the temperature of your food before you buy it, there are things you *can* do. Shop at a store you trust—one that buys from reputable sources. Once you purchase the food, it becomes your job to control the temperature at which it is kept. Don't leave the food sitting in a hot car. Remember that animal proteins are most often the source of food poisoning—that means poultry, fish, meat, eggs, and unpasteurized cheeses. Refrigerate meats, poultry, and seafood immediately and use them within 2 days or quick-freeze them as soon as you get home from shopping. Frozen foods should be kept frozen, defrosted in the fridge (not on the counter), and used soon after thawing.

Obviously, foods can be contaminated before they are purchased. The CDC found that poor hygiene and unsafe food sources accounted for more than a fourth of the outbreaks of food poisoning. Is your supermarket as clean as you would like? Are the employees impeccable in their handling of seafood and meat? As the consumer, you have a choice. Don't buy or use bulging cans, outdated foods, or packaged foods with broken seals. (See Table 4.2 for tips on making wise food selections.) Avoid buying overripe produce. Are you sometimes tempted to buy from roadside vendors? Beware of shelled eggs sitting out in flats, unrefrigerated. Be equally wary when buying fish. It may look good, but who knows where it was caught or how clean the ice is. Trust your powers of observation and your intuition. It's not worth the risk of becoming sick.

Situation: Food Storage

Fact

The CDC has found that a primary cause of food poisoning is keeping food at the wrong temperature. This caused a third of all the outbreaks from 1988 to 1992.

Table 4.2   Avoiding Food Contamination

Food	Preventive efforts	Risk
Soft cheeses: Brie, blue-veined, Camembert, feta	Avoid consumption by infants, children, pregnant women, elders, and those with chronic illness	Listeria
Fruit juices, cider	Buy pasteurized or bring to a boil	E. coli
Honey	Do not feed to infants or those who are immunocompromised	Botulism
Raw milk	To be safe, don't buy raw milk. Use only pasteurized dairy products	Campylobacter, E. coli, listeria, salmonella
Water	Buy bottled water or filter to "1-micron absolute," or boil for 15 minutes	Campylobacter, cryptosporidium, E. coli, giardia

SOURCE: FDA. Organisms that can bug you. *FDA Consumer.* 1991, Jan.–Feb.; revised 12/97, 11/00. Web site: www.cfsan.fda.gov/~dms/unwelcom.html.

Shopping Checklist

- Read labels to minimize the risk of food poisoning. Check the product date for freshness.
- Buy only milk and cheese products that are pasteurized. Anyone with compromised immunity should avoid unpasteurized cheeses such as Brie, Camembert, and blue-veined cheeses (to prevent listeria).
- Don't buy eggs that are unrefrigerated, for example, eggs sitting out at roadside stands (to prevent salmonella). And be sure to put

Shopping Checklist *(continued)*

eggs in the refrigerator once you get home.
(The FDA found that just keeping eggs cold
enough cut levels of bacteria by 25 percent.)

- Avoid prepared foods that contain raw or partially
  cooked meat or dairy products.
- Avoid potatoes that are green-skinned or have
  developed eyes and sprouts.
- Bag all vegetables before going through the
  checkout to avoid bacteria on the checkout
  counters.
- Put protein foods (chicken, fish, meat, and eggs)
  into plastic bags to prevent leakage of uncooked
  meat juices onto other foods, which causes cross
  contamination, the transmission of bacteria from
  one food to another.
- Avoid potentially contaminated foods: Don't buy
  food in damaged packaging; don't select food
  from unsafe displays such as those that feature
  cooked and uncooked seafood on the same bed
  of ice; don't accept free samples; avoid food from
  open-air displays of perishable food and from
  salad bars; don't purchase foods in stores with
  unsanitary conditions.
- Put chilled or frozen items, particularly any
  proteins, in the shopping cart last—right before
  you head for the checkout line.
- When loading the car, keep perishables inside
  the air-conditioned car, not the trunk.
- If you live more than a half an hour from the

store, bring an ice chest for storing perishables on the way home.

- Refrigerate or freeze perishables immediately— keep the fridge at 40°F and freezer at 0°F.
- Remember that chicken and fish need to be cooked the first or second day. So on the holidays, if you must buy these foods ahead, purchase them frozen. Fresh, unfrozen turkey needs to be bought just a day or two before you use it.

Germs

Campylobacter, *E. coli*, listeria, salmonella, other types of bacteria, and various molds

Overview

It is vital to store foods properly in order to prevent spoilage and vulnerability to pests and to preserve the wholesomeness of food as long as possible. The key is to keep food organized and clean and to use the food you buy in a timely manner. Assess your shelves on a regular basis to stay current on food items that are perishable.

Cold Food Storage

Foods can spoil. It's a simple fact. Most fresh fruits and vegetables, depending on their ripeness and refrigeration, have to be used within a few days to a week or two. Fresh-cut meats, poultry, and fish, which are most easily contaminated by bacteria, must be refrigerated and used within 2 days, or they should be frozen immediately. Whole grains and beans store well because of their protective coverings; when free of insecticides, they can be kept indefinitely, or at least a year or two. Store them well in sealed containers to avoid insects. On the other hand, flours, which are ground grain, keep better in the refrigerator or freezer. Nuts and seeds are definitely best refrigerated or stored in the freezer because they contain oils and more easily become rancid. (See Table 4.3 for tips on cold food storage.)

Many foods that are prepackaged in boxes, cans, and jars contain some kind of spoilage retardants and do fairly well when stored in cupboards. However, opened packages of cereals, crackers, and other grain products should be sealed tight and used within the month or be refrigerated to protect them from insect infestation. This is especially important in the warmer months since the smell of grains will attract grain moths, mice, and other critters.

Table 4.3 Cold Food Storage

Product	In fridge, unopened	In fridge, opened	In freezer
Homemade casseroles			1–2 months
Homemade or deli salads: macaroni, egg, chicken, tuna		3–5 days	Do not freeze well
Prefrozen casseroles, TV dinners	Keep frozen until ready to eat		3–4 months
Vacuum-packed dinners	2 weeks	3–4 days	
Spices: paprika		Refrigerate [store cold to avoid risk of salmonella]	
Soups and stews		3–4 days	2–3 months

Table 4.3 *(continued)*

Product	In fridge, unopened	In fridge, opened	In freezer
Egg whites or egg substitutes	10 days	3 days	12 months
Fresh eggs in shell		3–5 weeks	Do not freeze well
Hard-boiled eggs		1 week	Do not freeze well
Cooked egg dishes		3–4 days	
Milk		5 days	1 month
Swiss, brick, processed cheese		3–4 weeks	Affects texture and taste
Whole, uncooked chicken,	1–2 days	1–2 days	12 months
Cooked chicken	3–4 days	3–4 days	4 months
Canned poultry	2–5 years	3–4 days	
Lean fish (such as cod)		1–2 days	Up to 6 months
Fatty fish (blues, perch, salmon)		1–2 days	2–3 months
Gravy		1–2 days	3 months
Hot dogs	2 weeks	1 week	1–2 months
Deli and lunch meats	2 weeks	3–5 days	Do not freeze well
Ground beef		1–2 days	3–4 months
Steaks and roasts		3–5 days	6–12 months
Pork chops		3–5 days	3–4 months
Roasts, uncooked sausage		1–2 days	1–2 months

SOURCES: Food and Drug Administration Web site, www.fda.gov from Food Marketing Institute for fish and dairy products, USDA for other foods. Adapted from FDA. The unwelcome dinner guest: Preventing foodborne illness. *FDA Consumer.* 1991, Jan.–Feb.; revised 12/97, 2/99, 10/99, and 6/00. On the FDA Web site: www.cfsan.fda.gov/~dms/qa-sto8.html.

Storing Perishables

- After shopping, unload perishables first and immediately refrigerate them.

- When storing dried foods and root vegetables, never store them directly under a sink, and always keep foods off the floor and separate from chemicals and cleaning supplies.
- You may want to wash your vegetables when you get them home. Store them at 40° Farenheit (5°C) or below.
- Wash your vegetables thoroughly to minimize the risk of contamination.
- To maximize freshness, keep vegetables in bags, and keep other foods in covered containers.
- Store eggs in their carton inside the fridge to keep them cold, rather than on the refrigerator door where it's warmer.
- Check the labels on condiments and other foods that need to be refrigerated once they're opened.
- Since animal proteins spoil the most easily of all foods, store securely wrapped packages of meat, poultry, or fish in the meat drawer or coldest section of the fridge. Be sure that juices don't drip and contaminate other foods. Immediately freeze any fish or poultry you're not going to cook within 2 days or meat you plan to keep longer than 3 to 5 days. You can keep meats and fish a little colder by placing a package of blue ice on top of the food.
- When storing leftovers, divide foods into shallow containers for rapid cooling. Slice foods such as egg dishes into serving-size pieces so the food will be thoroughly chilled.
- Use cooked leftovers within 4 days. If you want to be superorganized, you can keep labels and a pen in the kitchen and date leftovers.

- Periodically double-check the temperature of your fridge with an appliance thermometer. The temperature should be 40°F (about 5°C).

Frozen Foods

- You can freeze almost anything except canned foods and eggs in shells. Once food is out of the can, you can freeze it.
- Foods stored at 0°F are protected from the growth of microbes such as bacteria and molds, which enter a dormant state at very cold temperatures. However, once thawed, bacteria again become active and can multiply rapidly. So after the food is thawed, thoroughly cook it immediately to destroy any microbes.
- Check the temperature of your freezer or freezing compartment every so often, or keep a thermometer in it to make it easier to check more often. The temperature needs to be 0°F or below to assure safe storage.
- The FDA reports that freezing does not destroy nutrient content. Freezing does slow enzyme activity, for better and for worse. Partial cooking—blanching— is necessary to prepare foods for freezing.
- Freeze foods as rapidly as possible, ideally in 2 hours. Spread foods in a single layer and then stack them after they're frozen.
- Accidentally frozen cans may cause health problems. Discard them to be safe.
- If there's a power failure, keep the freezer door closed. A separate free-standing chest or upright freezer will

keep food frozen for 2 days if it's fully loaded. Add blue ice or dry ice to keep things cold until the power returns.

- You can protect against loss of frozen food by freezing gallon jugs of spring water. This provides extra refrigerant, should the power go out, and also large amounts of bottled water in case of emergency. Or use freezer gels—blue ice or dry ice—until the power returns.
- Perishable items can be refrozen if they still contain ice crystals or feel cold to the touch.
- Discard any food that is room temperature. But *don't* taste it—food may look and smell fine and yet still contain dangerous bacteria. *When in doubt, throw it out!*

Dry Food Storage

Storing Dry Foods Safely

- Some types of ceramic dinnerware have lead in the glaze:
  - Don't store acidic foods, such as fruit juices or tomato sauce, in ceramic containers.
  - Avoid the use of antique or collectible housewares for storing food and beverages.
  - Don't store beverages in lead crystal containers.
- Packaging on microwavable foods can contaminate the food when it is cooked at high temperatures. Discard the packaging and use only microwave-safe containers.

- Avoid storing food in cabinets under the sink or near water, drains or heating pipes. Food stored there can attract insects and rodents through the openings to the pipes.
- Clean the tops of cans before opening.
- Select your pots and pans with care. Stainless steel and glazed ironware appear to be the best choices. Avoid aluminum and also copper cookware until the last word is in on their toxicity. In the case of aluminum, it has been linked with Alzheimer's disease in several studies. See Table 4.4 for tips on dry food storage.

Table 4.4   Dry Food Storage

Food item	Storage time	Specifics
Canned fruits and vegetables	1 year	After opening, remove from can and refrigerate
Chocolate	18 months	Keep cool
Coffee	1 to 2 years in the can	Refrigerate or freeze
Dry milk (nonfat)	6 months	Keep in airtight container
Unbleached flour	8–12 months	
Whole wheat flour	3–6 months	Refrigerate whole wheat flour
Honey	1 year	Do not feed to young children
Mayonnaise and dressings	6–12 months	Keep in fridge no more than 3 months after opening
Molasses	6–12 months	Keep tightly covered

Table 4.4 (continued)

Food item	Storage time	Specifics
Vegetable oil	Estimates range	Store in fridge
Olive oil	from 6 weeks	Store in cool,
	to 3–6 months	dark place
Macaroni	1–2 years	Keep container
Egg noodles	6 months	airtight
Peanut butter	6–9 months	Can turn rancid when exposed to air or heat
White rice	1–2 years	Keep in airtight
Brown rice	6 months	container
Salad dressings	6–12 months	Keep in refrigerator 3 months
Whole spices	1–2 years	Heat and long-term
Ground herbs	6 months	storage can affect color and aroma

SOURCE. FDA. Safe Storage. Web site: www.cfsan.fda.gov/~dms/qa-sto9.html.

Avoiding Pests

- Never buy food in broken or opened packages. Once packages are opened at home, it's most ideal to transfer the contents to impenetrable jars or tins with tight-fitting lids. This is true of crackers, grains, and cereals, particularly if there is any kind of infestation already in the kitchen or anywhere in the house.
- If you find contamination, discard all prepared food in open packages. This includes opened or damaged packages of cereals, dried fruits, nuts, flour, meal, cornstarch, crackers, breakfast foods, dehydrated foods, macaroni, chocolate, cocoa, dry soup mixes, spices of all kinds, dry dog food, and birdseed.

- Clean the kitchen shelves and periodically clean all the nooks and corners of the kitchen. Pests are also more easily trapped in a clean kitchen since the bait becomes the main source of food.
- Limit the access of pests. Make sure window screens fit tightly. Plug holes in the wall that lead to the outside or, if you're in an apartment, that lead to other units. Holes can be sealed inexpensively with spackling compound. Large holes can be stuffed with steel wool and then spackled.
- Refrigerate foods such as ground grains even though they are traditionally stored dry. Although whole grains are remarkably stable for storage, ground grains in cereals and flours are much more subject to both pests and mold. Refrigeration limits the access of pests. However, it doesn't control mold unless the cereal or flour is in an airtight container.
- Take away the pests' food supply by keeping living areas clean. Be especially careful to sweep up food crumbs, wipe up spills when they happen, wash dishes immediately, and deposit leftover food in its proper place. Empty garbage cans frequently, and if necessary, accumulate garbage in a plastic bag with a twist tie to eliminate the enticing odors of decaying food.
- Dry up the pests' water supply. Repair leaky faucets, pipes, and clogged drains. Insects have to drink somewhere—don't let poor plumbing cause leaks that attract bugs.
- Get rid of any clutter that pests can hide in. Clean out your attic, basement, and closets—pests anywhere in the house may eventually find their way to the

kitchen. Remove piles of old clothing, newspapers, magazines, and boxes. Check out-of-the-way places where unused items often get tossed (for instance, under stairwells). See Table 4.5 for tips on protecting dry food from common pests.

Table 4.5   Common Pests—Stored Food

Pest	Concerns	Attractants	Solutions
Ants	Invasive pest; some species bite or sting; some can carry disease	Fatty, sweet, and protein foods (meats, peanut butter, fruit juice etc.); water	Destroy outside nests; sprinkle red chili pepper, paprika, dried peppermint, or borax; plant mint around the house
Beetles	Allergic reactions from breathing fragments; intestinal distress, lesions, and possible infection from ingesting larvae	Grains, cereals, other grain products, dried fruits, sweets, spices; some infest meat, fish, cheese; cat and dog food	Good hygiene; use tight-fitting #30-mesh screens on doors; check packaged foods before you bring them home; store food in containers, avoid moldy foods; cook meats thoroughly
Cockroaches	Possible transmission of salmonella, toxoplasmosis, or other microbes; may cause allergies	Bags, cartons, any human or animal food; water; the insides of TVs, alarm clocks, radios, even refrigerators!	Good house-keeping: don't leave food out overnight; use boric acid; an electronic roach zapper or jar traps

Table 4.5 *(continued)*

Pest	Concerns	Attractants	Solutions
Flies	Possible transmission of cholera and typhoid, intestinal worms, poliovirus, salmonella, shigella	All foods; garbage, lawn clippings, any other kind of decaying matter	Remove garbage promptly; use tight-fitting screens on windows; eliminate food sources; hang clusters of cloves; employ citrus oil aromatherapy; use flypaper
Mites	Dermatitis	Products high in fat such as peanuts, cheese, and ham; sweets; grains	Refrigerate foods; use sealed containers
Moths	Avoid ingesting larvae	Flour, cereal, biscuits, nuts, dried fruit, chocolate, dog food	Replace staples frequently; store in closed containers; refrigerate flours; discard any "webby" food; sift flours (#64 mesh)
Rats and mice	Can carry insects and disease	Attracted to food garbage; may infest walls of homes	Get a cat; use mousetraps baited with peanut butter; nontoxic repellents and traps

SOURCES: Information sources include Debra Dadd-Redalia, *Home Safe Home.* New York: J.P. Tarcher, 1997. www.DLD123.com; Walter Ebeling. *Urban Entomology.* Web site www.entomology.ucr.edu/ebeling/; *Whatever Works Catalogue* [Pest Control Products]. Web site at www.whateverworks.com; and others.

Situation: Food Preparation

Fact

The majority of food poisoning comes from just two main sources: protein foods that have not been fully cooked and vegetables that have not been adequately washed.

Sources of Exposure

- Protein foods—rare or raw meat, fish, uncooked eggs, raw milk
- Vegetables that are not adequately washed

Germs

Any of the germs that cause food poisoning, especially *E. coli*, salmonella, and campylobacter

Overview

It is essential that all those who handle food wash their hands conscientiously and avoid handling foods when they are sick. People with cuts or open sores on their hands should wear rubber gloves to reduce the spread of bacteria. Be sure to wash your hands before working with food, especially after handling money or animals. It's also important to wash your hands while caring for children, particularly after wiping noses or changing diapers. In these situations, you'll want to wash your hands with antibacterial soap and clean your nails with a brush and soap or hydrogen peroxide.

Impeccable food handling takes a little planning. For example, it takes between 5 and 20 minutes to presoak salad vegetables. If you decide to use this extra step in cleaning the vegetables that you don't cook, that needs to be built into your routine either when you first come home from the store or before you prepare the evening meal.

Cooking Safety

Cooking temperatures: One of the primary reasons we cook food is to sanitize it. Remember that heat kills bacteria. But it has to be hot enough—160 to 180°F.

Cooking times: It has been suggested that you cook all meat, chicken, and fish at least 20 minutes, until all portions of the food are well done.

Meats, Poultry, and Fish

- Marinate meat and poultry in a covered dish *in the fridge.*
- Don't interrupt the cooking process. Never refrigerate partially cooked products.
- Thaw foods in the fridge rather than on the counter. This can take some planning—a 20-pound turkey needs 4 days to thaw in the refrigerator!
- Frozen foods can also be thawed by submerging them in cold tap water. You need to protect the food by placing it in a sealed plastic bag. Be sure to change the water every 30 minutes so the food won't get too warm, and make sure the bag doesn't leak.
- Thaw foods thoroughly, so they can cook all the way through.

- Use a meat thermometer to be sure protein foods are thoroughly cooked—it could save your life!
- Use a conventional meat thermometer. It gives you more information than a pop-up thermometer.
- Cook all meats until well done, with no pink (except turkey and smoked meats, which will continue to appear pink despite their temperature). To ensure that foods are well done, make sure they register 160 to 170°F on the thermometer. Juices should run clear, not red.
- If you're making stuffing, cook it separately from the chicken or turkey, on the stovetop or in the oven. If you must cook it inside, stuff the turkey just before baking, and make sure the stuffing reaches 165°F on the thermometer.

For more information on safe cooking temperatures, see Table 4.6.

Table 4.6   Safe Cooking Temperatures

Food	Temperature	Risk
Uncooked eggs in any form—for example, eggnog, lightly cooked eggs in omelets, French toast, Caesar salad, hollandaise sauce, mousse, meringue pie, quiche	Cook to 160°F—until no longer runny Scrambled eggs—1 minute (250°F) Sunny-side up—7 minutes or 4 minutes covered Fried—3 minutes first side, 1 minute other side Poached—5 minutes in boiling water Boiled—7 minutes in boiling water	Listeria, salmonella

Table 4.6 *(continued)*

Food	Temperature	Risk
Raw cheeses: Brie, blue-veined, Camembert, feta	To be avoided by infants, children, pregnant women, elders, and those with chronic illness	Listeria
Raw milk	Pasteurize	Campylobacter, *E. coli*, listeria, salmonella
Beef, veal, lamb	Avoid all raw meats	*E. coli*, listeria, salmonella
Ground beef, ham	160°	
Meats, medium done	160°	
Meats, well done	170°	
Pork	Cook to 160°–170°	Listeria, trichinosis
Ham	Cook at 160°; if the ham is precooked, cook at 140°	
Uncooked poultry		
Ground chicken or turkey	165°	
Whole chicken or turkey	180°	
Breasts, roasts	170°	
Thighs, wings	Cook until juices run clear	Cyclospora, campylobacter, listeria, salmonella
Fish	Cook well; should be flaky, not rubbery, when cut	Botulism
Raw seafood	Note source of seafood; cook seafood well; avoid sushi, sashimi	Cholera, listeria, staph, vibrio
Shellfish: clams, cockles, mussels, oysters, scallops	Raw seafood should not be eaten. Cook well; avoid lightly steamed seafood	Hepatitis A
Leftovers	165°F; meats in 200°F oven; warming tray 140°F	Any bacteria
Home-canned foods	Before eating, boil for 10 minutes at above 165°F	Botulism

Source: Adapted from FDA. The unwelcome dinner guest: Preventing foodborne illness. *FDA Consumer.* 1991, Jan.–Feb.; revised 12/97, 2/99, 10/99, and 6/00. FDA Web site: www.cfsan.fda.gov/~dms/fdunwelc.html.

Eggs and Egg Dishes

- Never eat raw eggs or foods that contain them (to avoid salmonella).
- Use pasteurized eggs in place of raw eggs to make homemade ice cream, eggnog, Caesar salad, mayonnaise, and hollandaise sauce. Commercial versions of these products are okay because they're made with pasteurized liquid eggs.
- If you want to pasteurize the eggs yourself, heat the egg-milk mixture to 160°F (until it coats a metal spoon). When you don't have time to make or buy pasteurized eggs, leave them out of the recipe rather than take a chance.
- Don't eat cookie dough that contains uncooked eggs. (If you find the dough irresistible, make or buy pasteurized eggs for the batter.)
- Eating foods made with eggs that are lightly cooked, such as French toast or meringue, can also be risky. Consider making these dishes with pasteurized eggs.
- Keep eggs in the fridge below 40°F. Cook them at 140°F or hotter.
- When cooking eggs, make sure the yolk and white are firm, not runny. Eggs need to be cooked on both sides, rather than just sunny-side up. Cook scrambled eggs until firm. (If you're served runny eggs in a restaurant, send them back—*it's your health!*)
- Avoid keeping raw or cooked eggs or egg dishes out of the fridge for more than 2 hours. Even Easter eggs should be refrigerated after 2 hours or considered not for eating—for decoration only.

- When refrigerating a dish made with eggs, divide it and store it in several shallow containers so it will cool throughout.

Defrosting

- Three of the safest ways to defrost foods are in the fridge; in the sink, in cold water; and in the microwave.
- Plan ahead for slow, safe thawing, figuring that it will probably take a day or two.
- For faster defrosting, place food in a leakproof plastic bag and immerse it in cold water. Change the water every 30 minutes and then immediately refrigerate the food.
- When defrosting food in the microwave, plan to cook it immediately. Some areas of the food may begin to cook during microwaving, activating bacteria— cooking it right away destroys the bacteria.
- Once food has been thawed in the fridge, it is safe to refreeze it without cooking. Cooked foods can also be frozen. But it's important to keep them either very hot or very cold.

Leftovers and Convenience Foods

- Don't taste food to be sure it's still good. There may be no sign that it's spoiled even though it is.
- If a food does taste or smell spoiled, take it back to the store, or throw it out.
- If you're microwaving your food, follow the directions carefully. Since the goal is to cook protein foods thoroughly, be sure to include the "standing time"

that some microwave recipes include. This is also part of the cooking process.

- Reheat leftovers thoroughly to 165°F or until hot and steamy. Bring soups, sauces, and gravies to a rolling boil.
- Use leftovers within 3 to 4 days.

Preparing Salads and Vegetables

Cleaning Vegetables—Lowering Your Risks of Exposure to Germs and Chemicals

It is wise to wash all fresh food thoroughly, since about two-thirds of nonorganic food typically contains pesticide residues. In addition, any food could be contaminated with insects eggs or germs such as *E. coli* or cyclospora. When preparing nonorganic produce, the outer layer should be discarded. Peel fruits and strip the outer leaves of lettuces and leafy greens. Rather than just rinsing the outside of leafy vegetables, such as lettuce, for example, wash the leaves individually. Different agents are available for washing:

- *Hydrogen peroxide* in a water solution has gotten good press recently as an effective antibacterial agent that is also relatively benign. It has been suggested that it can be used to effectively wash vegetables that will not be cooked. Hydrogen peroxide has also been used in combination with vinegar to clean vegetables.
- *Produce washes* are available at health food stores. These are mild detergents that contain natural oils, used in a soak to remove additional surface contaminants. Most are not "disinfectants"—they are not proven to destroy microbes. Without actual

testing, it's difficult to know the strengths and limitations of any particular product.[2]

- *Vinegar is* sometimes proposed for washing vegetables. However, research on the disinfectant properties of vinegar found that it effectively destroyed some bacteria, but not others.
- A *solution of bleach* in water. Bleach has been evaluated by researchers for its antimicrobial properties as a vegetable wash. Although bleach is an effective disinfectant, there is limited information on its toxicity, so we cannot currently recommend it.[3–6]
- *Dish detergent* is sometimes recommended as a vegetable wash, but current thinking advises against it. Since small residues of the detergent probably cling to the produce, the concern here is that most dish detergents are not designed for human consumption and may contain chemicals, colors, and perfumes.

Serving Food Safely

Bacteria thrive in the same environments we do—at room temperature. So keep food very hot or very cold from kitchen to table.

- Serve cooked foods as soon as they come off the heat.
- To avoid bacteria, be sure not to leave food out longer than 2 hours.
- On a hot day, over 90°F, don't leave food out longer than 1 hour!
- When serving food at a buffet, keep hot food over a heat source and keep cold food on ice.

- Keep platters of food refrigerated until it's time to serve or heat them.
- Don't serve all the food at once. Keep the second and third servings hot (above 140°F) or cold in the fridge (below 40°F).
- As you serve later courses, put the food on clean platters, instead of adding it to platters that have been sitting out (because the bacteria build up on the plates at room temperature).
- On a picnic, carry perishable foods in a cooler with a cold pack or ice and keep them in the shade.
- Keep hot food hot! Keep cold food cold!

Situation: Kitchen Hygiene

Fact

The CDC found that poor hygiene and unsafe food sources account for more than one-fourth of all food poisoning outbreaks.

Fact

According to research at the University of Arizona[7] the average kitchen sponge holds more than 100,000 bacteria!

Germs

Exposure can result from several sources:

- Inadequate hand washing—after using the bathroom or diapering children

- Cross-contamination—handling raw meat, poultry, or seafood (protein foods) and then preparing salads or other foods that won't be cooked
- Countertops, cutting boards, and utensils contaminated by raw protein foods
- Kitchen surfaces contaminated by sponges or dish towels

Overview

It is essential that all the members of your household who handle food make sure they wash their hands thoroughly before every meal and avoid handling foods when they're sick. Again, hand-washing is essential before working with food, especially after going to the bathroom, handling money or animals, or caring for children.

Countertops, cutting boards, and other surfaces should be cleaned after each use so that organisms don't grow. Keep cutting utensils spotlessly clean. Avoid the use of sponges—instead, use paper towels for cleaning counters and use scubbing pads that you replace weekly for cleaning pots and pans. Can openers need to be cleaned often and replaced frequently. Pots and pans, blenders, juicers, and other appliances need to be thoroughly cleaned after each use. Read ahead for more tips on keeping food and kitchen areas sparkling clean.

Keeping a Clean Kitchen

- If you're sick, don't cook. Food handling is a major way that germs are spread. If you must cook, wear disposable gloves. Consider the use of convenience foods or carryout until you're better.

- Keep shelves, countertops, refrigerator, freezer, and utensils really clean.
- Wipe countertops with hot water and soap and then with a disinfectant—preferably a safe cleaner such as an antibacterial soap, hydrogen peroxide, or a diluted bleach solution.
- If you wash the dishes by hand, do them within 2 hours after they've been used. Don't let them soak— this creates a "bacterial soup."
- If you use a dishwasher, keep the water nice and hot. This is actually a very effective way to sterilize your dishes, but do them immediately. If they sit in the dishwasher overnight, they could be subject to bacteria or mold.
- Counters and utensils used to cook meat can be sanitized with a solution of 1 teaspoon of bleach in 1 quart of water.
- You can also clean the drain of the kitchen sink by pouring a bleach and water solution down the drain, using this same formula.
- Clean your kitchen equipment thoroughly. On holidays, when your are using equipment that has been stored, clean it before using it. (A nice way to prepare for the holiday is to thoroughly clean the house and the kitchen the weekend before. Then you are cooking in an environment that's both pleasing and hygienic.)
- Wash cloth dish towels on the hot water cycle—and wash them frequently. Avoid the use of sponges. Instead, use disposable, recycled paper towels and scrubbing pads that you change weekly or even more often.
- Wash your hands in soap and water for 20 seconds before and after handling food. *You'll find that*

20 seconds is an amazingly long time—but it's important!

- Be sure to wash up every time you change the baby, use the bathroom, or blow your nose.
- Wash thoroughly after handling pets, before you begin to cook. Animals harbor many germs that can be harmful to humans. Reptiles and turtles can transmit salmonella and listeria. Cats may carry *H. pylori* bacteria (one of the major causes of ulcers) and toxoplasmosis (devastating to the unborn).
- Be sure to keep cats and other animals off the table and the counters.
- After using the bathroom, scrub under your nails with a brush dipped in hydrogen peroxide. That can prevent the transfer of bacteria or microscopic parasites, which tend to lodge under the fingernails.
- Avoid cross-contamination. Wash up after handling one food and before preparing the next—this is especially important if you are handling raw protein such as chicken, fish, meat, or eggs. It also minimizes the contamination of other foods that won't be cooked, such as salads.
- Ideally have two cutting boards—one for meat and the other for vegetables. Save wooden boards made of hard maple for use with salads and vegetables.
- Use plastic cutting boards for preparing protein foods (chicken, fish, and meat). Research has shown that plastic boards collect less bacteria and are more easily cleaned than wooden cutting boards. Replace the plastic boards when they become scored by knife abrasion, since bacteria can collect on the uneven surface.
- Be sure to clean all cutting boards with soap, hot water, and a bleach solution (1 teaspoon of bleach to a

quart of hot water). Soak the surface for several minutes and then dry it thoroughly. Or wash the cutting board in the dishwasher (For more suggestions, see Table 4.7.)

Table 4.7   Cleaning Products

Product	Concerns	Best option
Dish washing liquid	May have dye, chlorine, artificial fragrance	"Green" products
Dishwasher powder	Chlorine	"Green" products
Cleanser	Chlorine; possible asbestos in cleanser	Nonchlorinated scouring powder; baking soda, borax, table salt
Germ-killing disinfectants	Cresol, phenol, ethanol, formaldehyde, ammonia, chlorine	½ cup borax in 1 gallon hot water; aqueous solution of benzalkonium chloride; hydrogen peroxide; and vinegar; Oxyclean for bleach
Drain cleaners	Lye (poisonous)	1 handful baking soda and ½ cup white vinegar or ½ cup each salt and baking soda followed by hot water. Then clean the drain with a plunger
Ammonia and all-purpose cleaners	Ammonia (skin irritant, possible chemical burns); aerosol sprays	1 quart hot water in a spray bottle or bucket with either liquid soap or borax; or green products
Cleaners for appliances		½ teaspoon washing soda, 2 teaspoons liquid soap, and 2 cups hot water

Table 4.7 (continued)

Product	Concerns	Best option
Oven cleaner	Lye, ammonia, aerosols	Use 2 tablespoons liquid soap, 2 tablespoons borax, and warm water; for really dirty ovens, use chemical cleaners carefully, in a spray bottle
Glass cleaners	Ammonia, blue dye, aerosols	Solution consisting of half water and half vinegar in spray bottle or bucket
Mold and mildew cleaners	Kerosene, formaldehyde, phenol, pentachlorophenol	Clean with borax or vinegar and water. Reduce the level of moisture by keeping the area warmer or using a dehumidifier.

SOURCES: Debra Dadd-Redalia, *Home Safe Home.* New York: J. P. Tarcher, 1997. Web site www.DLD123.com, and other sources.

Situation: Packing Healthy Lunches and Snacks

Fact

On a hot day when the temperature is 90° or higher, bacteria in food can double their number every 20 minutes. Even the most nutritious packed lunches can contain bacteria that could cause illness. Bacteria thrive in warm, moist foods. They grow at temperatures between 40 and 140°F—above freezing and a little below boiling.

The growth of bacteria also depends on the moisture content and the acidity of the food. Bacteria tend to thrive in protein foods such as eggs, milk, meat, fish, and poultry. There are two main ways to make a packed lunch safer:

- Choose foods that can be kept safely at room temperature.
- Keep the bacteria count low by keeping cold foods very cold (on ice) and hot foods hot (in a thermos).

Keeping Cold Foods Cold

There are several practical ways to keep perishable foods cold. You can:

- Use a refreezable gel pack.
- Use thermoses or containers with a lid that can be frozen.
- Freeze juice in boxes or cans and then pack the juice with the lunch. The juice thaws and is ready to drink in 3 to 4 hours and the rest of the lunch has been kept cool.
- Freeze bottled spring water.
- Freeze sandwiches using hearty bread that will hold up well.

Pack it in an insulated lunch box. Metal or plastic lunch boxes can also be used. If lunch is carried in paper bags, double-bagging will also help to insulate food better. An ice source should be packed with perishable food in any type of lunch. Pack the container with enough gel packs or containers of frozen juice or bottled water to keep the food very cold, at 40°F. Pack food right from the refrigerator or freezer into the lunch container. When taking a lunch to work, obviously if there is a refrigerator, store perishable items there on arrival.

In the classroom, packed lunches should be kept out of direct sunlight and away from radiators, baseboards, and other heat sources. Take a few minutes to role-play these scenarios with younger children—ask them to find the coolest places where they might stow their lunch. Once gel packs and other cold sources melt, perishable foods are not safe—and should be tossed immediately. It's not worth taking the chance of getting sick.

Lunch Prep

- **Cold foods.** It's a good idea to prepare the food the night before. Freeze sandwiches, juice or water, and blue ice or thermos lids. Store everything except dried foods in the refrigerator. Make sandwiches with cold ingredients—freeze or chill the bread and chill the sandwich filling before assembling. Room-temperature bread can warm up any of the ingredients, making them subject to spoilage.

In the morning, pack the lunch container with sandwiches, fruit, and vegetables. Lettuce and tomatoes can be packed separately and added at lunchtime since they don't freeze well. Or you can send easy-to-eat chunky salads made without lettuce, served in a thermos. Another option is vegetables that can be eaten as finger food. Last, add cookies, granola, and other items that shouldn't be refrigerated. Then, place the ice pack(s) in the lunch box.

- **Hot foods.** Use an insulated bottle to keep hot foods hot. Fill the bottle with boiling water and let it stand for a few minutes. Heat the soup very hot before filling the thermos.

• **No waste.** Pack just the amount of perishable food that can be eaten at lunch. That way, you won't have to worry about the safety of leftovers. Discard any protein or dairy items left in the lunch box at the end of the day. Wash the lunch box daily with soap and water. Wash it weekly with baking soda to prevent odors.

Good Choices

Giving school-aged kids a say in their lunch menu boosts the odds that they will actually eat what you send. Plan the lunch menu with your children. Have them help prepare the lunch. Kids like small things, so pack portions that are kid-size. Make lunches fun—be creative. Take your children shopping, teach them how to read food labels, and coach them in how to select nutritious foods for their lunch. (See the Resources section at the end of the book for books on good nutrition.)

Stable Foods

Some food is safe without a cold source. Foods that can safely be left at room temperature for 4 to 6 hours include:

- Fresh fruit such as apples, peaches, ripe plums, and tangerines (other fruits, such as melons, oranges, pineapple, and kiwi, are less messy if they're cut up and carried in a small container).
- Nuts, peanuts, pumpkin and sunflower seeds, trail mix.
- Peanut butter sandwiches (try almond butter for a treat).
- Dry or hard cheeses, string cheese, and cheese sticks such as mozzarella.

- Yogurt in many forms, including drinkables; most yogurts can also be frozen.
- Canned fish, such as salmon, in cans that can be opened easily (with pull-tabs). Once the can is open, the contents should be eaten immediately. We now advise against consuming canned tuna on a regular basis. Recent research has shown that canned tuna is often laden with mercury, so we can no longer recommend it as a staple in the diet.
- Fresh, raw vegetables such as carrots, sweet red or green pepper strips, jicima, hearts of celery, or romaine lettuce.
- Chunky salads made of any of the ingredients above, or fresh tomatoes and cucumber.
- Breads, especially whole-grain breads, rolls, and crackers; bagels; pita bread; muffins; English muffins
- Chips, popcorn
- Dry whole-grain cereals
- Butter; cooking oil in dressings, such as olive oil
- Pickles, relish, mustard, and ketchup
- Snack-type puddings, as long as they're not too sweet; these can also be frozen.

Perishables

Cold Foods

As a general rule, if a food must be kept in the refrigerator, it is not safe for school lunches unless it can be kept very cold. Examples include meat, dairy products, eggs, seafood, cooked leftovers, and cooked vegetables and entrees. The foods that are most important to keep cold are proteins—chicken, turkey, lean luncheon meats, fish, and eggs—since they are highly perishable.

- *Prepackaged combos* may also need to be kept refrigerated—especially those that contain luncheon meats along with crackers, cheese, and condiments. This is important even if the luncheon meat or smoked ham has been cured or contains preservatives.
- *Home-cooked meats* used in sandwiches should be cooled quickly after being cooked and should be kept refrigerated until the sandwich is made. Use a fork, spatula, or tongs to place meat, poultry, or fish in the sandwich. This will prevent the spread of bacteria from fingers to food.[8]

Foods That Need to Be Kept Very Cold

Prepare cooked food ahead of time to allow for thorough chilling in the refrigerator, particularly turkey, ham, chicken, and vegetable or pasta salads. Divide large amounts of food into shallow containers for faster chilling and easier use. Keep cooked food refrigerated until it's time to leave home. Foods that should be frozen, kept cold with a refreezable ice pack, or stored in a thermos with a freezer lid include:

- *Sandwiches and salads* that contain meat, fish, or poultry
- *Custards and puddings* that are not prepackaged and any other foods that contain eggs
- *Milk and milk products* unless they have been vacuum-packed (except hard cheeses and yogurt)
- *Processed meats* (bologna, hot dogs, ham, etc.)

Note that sandwiches tend to freeze well if they are frozen in the thicker plastic bags designed for this purpose. (Avoid using thin sandwich bags.) You'll probably find that some breads freeze better than others.

To prepare frozen sandwiches, spread each piece of bread from edge to edge with a natural mayonnaise from the health food store. This can keep the bread from absorbing moisture. Sandwiches can be kept frozen for 3 to 4 weeks. Although commercial natural mayonnaise is not as volatile as homemade mayo, all mayonnaise-based salads with ingredients such as tuna, salmon, chicken, or eggs should be kept very cold. The use of homemade mayonnaise containing raw eggs is never recommended since eggs must be cooked thoroughly to guard against salmonella. Although butter could be used as a spread, one must recognize that butter is also made up of saturated fats, which have adverse effects in the body. These "bad" fats are known to affect fatty acid metabolism and cholesterol levels, and therefore we would not recommend their use on a regular basis.

One or two sandwiches will thaw in about 3 to 3½ hours. In preparing sandwiches, keep these tips in mind:

- Sandwich fillings that freeze well include cheddar cheese or cream cheese, sliced or ground meat, sliced or ground poultry, fish, and cooked egg yolks.
- Fillings that do not freeze well include raw vegetables such as lettuce, carrots, or tomatoes, and those with egg whites, jelly, or mayonnaise. The vegetables become limp, the egg whites become tough, and the other fillings make the sandwich soggy.

In addition, when adding dessert, be aware that *homemade or deli custards, puddings, and cream pies* are so easily spoiled by bacteria that they should never be used in packed lunches unless they are kept cold by ice or refrigeration. They are available in prepackaged form although many tend to be overly sweetened.

Hot Dishes

Use an insulated container to keep foods such as soup, chili, and stew hot. Fill the container with boiling water, let it stand for a few minutes, empty it, and then pour the food in while it's piping hot. The insulated container needs to be kept closed until lunchtime to keep the food hot at 140°F or above. (If you have access to a kitchen at work, canned versions of these foods can be carried and heated.)

Other foods that should be kept hot in a thermos include:

- Cooked vegetables
- Cooked grains such as rice
- Dressings and gravies

When using the microwave oven to reheat lunches, cover the food to retain the moisture and promote safe, even heating. Reheat leftovers to at least 165°F. Food should be steaming hot. Cook frozen convenience meals according to the instructions on the package.

Takeout Lunches

If you're planning to get takeout foods such as fried chicken or barbecued beef, the rule of thumb used to be to eat takeout foods within 2 hours of pickup. Recent guidelines suggest that it's best to either eat foods immediately or refrigerate them right away.

It's important to help your children become aware of the necessity of safe food handling. A study of children in 4-H programs found that most of them were not knowledgeable about how or why to wash to wash their hands, why cold foods need to be kept cold, how foods packed in a lunch could be kept cold, or how to identify unsafe foods. The study found only about 33 percent washed their hands every time they packed their lunch, and only 41 percent washed them each time before eating at school. Training sessions in their groups improved these habits. Still, it is clear that we need to begin teaching these skills to our younger children, so that they become second nature.

Restaurants

Fact

The CDC estimates that more than 76 million cases of food-borne illness occur each year.[9] It is estimated that only 1 in every 25 to 100 cases requires medical attention.

Please take the possibility of food poisoning very seriously when you dine out. Food poisoning is uncomfortable, and it can be fatal. In your own home, you have some control—you know that you have kept the kitchen clean, that you have avoided cross-contamination when handling your food, and that you have cooked meats and poultry well.

When you dine out, you have limited control. What you *can* do is form a general impression of the cleanliness and con-scientiousness of the restaurant—and then exercise conscious choice about whether you will eat there or not. We don't want to be fatalistic, but it's important to remember that food poisoning can have very serious consequences, particularly for children, women who are pregnant, and others who are more vulnerable.

Selecting a Restaurant

- Take note of the general cleanliness and appearance of the restaurant. Mealtime is not a time to focus on picturesque qualities—but rather the aesthetics of cleanliness.
- How neat and clean are the waiters and waitresses? Is cleanliness a high priority to this establishment?
- If in doubt, ask to use the rest room before you decide to sit down and order. The state of the rest room is often a reflection of other areas behind the scenes, like the kitchen.
- Select restaurants with a good reputation. Is the restaurant recommended in a guidebook or in a recent newspaper clipping featured in the window?
- At mealtime, is the restaurant crowded? (If so, this is usually a good sign.) Do the locals eat there?
- If you're traveling and have time to plan ahead, you may want to check the web for restaurant ratings. At least two major cities post lists of restaurants that have been cited for health violations. Both New York and Los Angeles list eating establishments in violation on the web.

Ordering

- Eating raw or rare meat increases the risk of bacteria and parasites. Avoid foods such as rare steak or hamburger, beefsteak tartare, or pâté. (Risks include a highly toxic form of *E. coli* and campylobacter.)
- We face a number of choices when we consider dining on raw foods. Sushi, for example, is a relatively

low-calorie protein food that provides a pleasant dining experience. On the other hand, the incidence of various parasites has been associated with the consumption of sushi, as reported in the medical literature. Occasionally adults indulge in sushi, but it is important not to give children sushi that contains raw fish. California roll, for example, can be made with avocado, cooked sea leg, and rice. Another good choice is vegetarian sushi, which does not contain raw fish and therefore has no risk. These rolls are made with rice and avocado, cucumber, or other vegetables. These alternatives enable you to enjoy this cuisine without the concurrent risks.

- Avoid the salad bar, buffets, and other food displays that are exposed to airborne bacteria and the germs of other customers. Doctors report that eating in salad bars is a high-risk factor for parasites.
- When ordering egg dishes, have fried eggs cooked on both sides. Eggs that are only cooked on one side— sunny-side up—are not cooked sufficiently to destroy bacteria. Scrambled eggs should be cooked through until they are not runny.
- Do not eat foods containing raw or lightly cooked eggs, such as fresh Caesar salad dressing, hollandaise sauce, unpasteurized eggnog, souffles, meringues, and other desserts such as tirimisu. (Uncooked or unpasteurized eggs carry a risk of salmonella.)
- *Cautions for pregnant women, young children, the elderly, and those who are immunocompromised:* Just as you would at home, avoid raw or unpasteurized cheeses or milk, as well as lightly cooked foods made from them.

Once Your Food Is Served

- Make sure the food is served at the proper temperature—cold foods such as salads should be definitely cold, and hot foods should be hot.
- Check to be sure that beef, pork, and other meat and poultry dishes are well cooked. If meat is served pink or bloody, politely send it back to the kitchen for more cooking. Fish should be flaky, not rubbery, when cooked to the proper "doneness."
- Don't drink with your meal—water dilutes your stomach acid. *This acid is your primary protection against bad bugs and food poisoning.*
- You can also maintain good levels of protective stomach acid by avoiding the use of antacids.

Take encouragement from the fact that more than 54 billion meals are prepared and eaten outside the home each year. This means that many thousands of safe meals are served for every meal that causes a problem. In that context, trust your observations and your intuition, make wise choices, and enjoy.

5

Clean Drinking Water

Just as we want our food to be fresh, clean, and nutritious, the water we drink should be as clean and uncontaminated. Since water is second in importance only to the air we need for sustaining life, we don't want our water laced with toxins—germs or industrial chemicals.

Research by the Environmental Working Group in 1995 found that over 45 million Americans were supplied with tap water that failed to meet basic health standards.[1] A similar study in 1994 found that more than 53 million Americans drank water that did not meet the standards in the Safe Water Drinking Act. Federal and state records also show that the most frequent water problems occur due to microbes, particularly bacteria, such as *E. coli*, and parasites, such as giardia, which affect the water supply of at least 35 million people. And numerous city water systems have been found to harbor parasites such as giardia and cryptosporidium. Since five out of every six Americans use public water systems, this represents a major public health concern.

Our primary water problems include contamination from a wide variety of microbes (see Table 5.1), as well as industrial toxic wastes and agricultural chemicals. Bacteria, viruses, and

Table 5.1 Primary Sources of Waterborne Illness

Infectious illnesses	Number of reported cases, year 2000
Salmonella infections	41,901
Viral hepatitis A (from food or water)	30,021
Shigella infection	23,117
Cryptosporidium infections	3,128
Hemorrhagic *E. coli*	2,555

SOURCE: Data from CDC. Summary of Notifiable Diseases—United States, 2000. Morbidity and Mortality Weekly Report. 2002, June 14; 49 (53): 1–102.

protozoa can enter drinking water from human sewage or animal waste. Microbes cause diseases ranging from dysentery and hepatitis to Legionnaires' disease; *E. coli* alone sickens close to a million people a year, killing hundreds, including children. Waterborne microbes can cause infection in several ways:

1. **Waterborne infections**. These infections can be contracted by:
    - Drinking contaminated water or beverages with contaminated ice
    - Eating food that was washed or irrigated with contaminated water, or food that came in contact with contaminated ice
    - Coming into physical contact with contaminated water while bathing, performing occupational activities, swimming, or participating in water sports

2. **Infections carried by fish, shellfish, or other aquatic organisms.** For example, bacteria-laden oysters can cause cholera or other types of infection.

3. **Infections spread by insects that live on the water.**
   These infectious illnesses include encephalitis,
   caused by the West Nile virus, and malaria, caused
   by protozoa.

Many of these diseases can later be transmitted in
other ways, such as by person-to-person contact or through food
handling.

These microbes can produce symptoms that include mild
to life-threatening gastroenteritis, hepatitis, skin infections,
wound infections, and conjunctivitis, as well as respiratory or
generalized infection. Other microbes that can be transmitted
in water include enterovirus, francisella (which causes tularemia), hepatovirus (which causes hepatitis), and legionella
(which causes Legionnaires' disease). Two of the worst offend-
ers are giardia and cryptosporidium (both protozoa—microscopic parasites), which can cause severe cramping and
diarrhea, and can lead to dehydration or chronic GI illness if
they go undiagnosed.

At one time, we viewed water contamination by microbes
as a problem of Third World countries and other areas that do
not treat their water. But microbial outbreaks in the last 30 years
have taught us that these problems are universal. In Milwaukee
several years ago, more than 100 people died and more than
4000 were hospitalized from cryptosporidium in the city tap
water. In total, over 400,000 people were affected. Between
1971 and 1985, more than 100,000 cases of disease in the United
States were attributed to drinking water. Recently, the Centers
for Disease Control and the EPA advised individuals with a
compromised immune system to consult their physician before
drinking ordinary tap water!

Choosing Safe Drinking Water

At this point, the best solutions appear to be buying bottled water or filtering your drinking water. Options include bottled springwater collected from mountain or underground sources and filtered water from the tap or from a well. Even the purity of these resources periodically comes into question.

Tap Water

Most tap water comes either from surface reservoirs formed from rivers, streams, and lakes or from groundwater. Groundwater refers to the subterranean reservoirs that hold much of the earth's water and supply nearly all the rural drinking water and about half of city water supplies. The water from these sources goes through local treatment plants; many use a very old process involving settling tanks, filtration through sand and gravel, and then chemicals to clean up the water so it's fit for human use.

Numerous chemicals and minerals are used for "purification," including chlorine, alum or sodium aluminum salts, soda, ash, phosphates, calcium hydroxide, and activated carbon. Yet this process may not clear all the many environmental pollutants that can contaminate our water supplies, including animal wastes, fertilizers, herbicides, insecticides, petroleum products, chemicals, and toxic industrial wastes, including lead and radon. Much of this pollution affects not only surface waters, but also the groundwater in natural aquifers deep under the earth. As a result, most artesian well drinking waters are contaminated to a certain degree. Areas of greatest concern include microbial and lead contamination. City water is also heavily chlorinated to kill germs, and is fluoridated to prevent tooth decay. It may contain other additives. Many doctors now encourage their patients to use only purified drinking water and avoid tap water.

Information on the Water Quality in Your Area

Data can be obtained from municipal water districts and from the web site of the Environmental Working Group (www.ewg.org) or from the online Chemical Scorecard of the Environmental Defense Fund (www.scorecard.org). It is fairly inexpensive to have the bacteria count of your water verified, although this will not reflect contamination by other microbes, such as protozoa.

Making Tap Water Safer

Although chlorine is currently the most effective water disinfectant we have, it does not kill protozoa. Of particular importance are giardia and cryptosporidium, which can be fatal to AIDS patients, older people, and others who have vulnerable immune systems. Individuals with HIV will want to use bottled water or a tapwater filtration system that removes particles of 1 micron or larger. Those who wish to drink tap water are urged to boil it before drinking it to prevent microbial infections.

The most effective way to kill waterborne germs is to boil the water. Some sources recommend boiling for 1 minute. However, to be sure you've killed all the bacteria and viruses in the water, maintain the water at a full boil for at least 15 minutes. Add 5 minutes to the boiling time for every 1000 feet you are above sea level.

Well Water

Well water comes primarily from groundwater supplies and can vary greatly in its mineral content: Some are low in minerals, while others are a rich source of beneficial nutrients such as iron, zinc, selenium, magnesium, or calcium. Unfortunately, well water is not necessarily safe from contamination by microbes or chemicals, especially if you live in an agricultural area. Even if you have been using a particular well for a number of years, it is necessary to have the water checked for bacteria, parasites, chemicals, and minerals—your life could depend on it. With a clean bill of health and periodic testing, you will have greater peace of mind when you use the water. (See the Resources section at the end of the book for a list of companies that provide water testing.)

Bottled Water

At least one in six Americans uses some type of bottled water as the main source of drinking water. Bottled products include domestic and international springwaters, mineral waters, designer waters, flavored waters, juice waters, and others. Many are bottled from various artesian wells and natural underground springs from around the world. Bottled water is more likely to be clear of bacteria and toxic chemicals, but it too can come from contaminated groundwater. In some cases, these products have proved to be just filtered city tap water. When electing to have bottle water delivered, it seems appropriate to request test results from the bottler. Ideally, the company can provide reports from independent lab testing, that is performed regularly.

Springwater

This is the "natural" water found in surface or underground springs. It may be filtered or disinfected with chlorine, but otherwise it is not usually processed. However, some spring-water is bottled at the source, while other springwaters are transported and then treated and bottled. (Water bottled at the source is preferable.) Just as groundwater can be polluted, springwater can also be contaminated. Although springwater can be costly in general, it's high on the list of drinkable waters. Excellent bottled waters are available that have been distilled, filtered, or spring-fed, including a variety of waters from around the world.

Mineral Water

Essentially, most waters are mineral waters—that is, they contain minerals. For example, in California, the standard for bottled mineral water is more than 500 parts per million (ppm) of dissolved minerals. Underground bubbly water, called "natural sparkling water," usually contains lots of minerals, as well as carbon dioxide (CO_2). Many companies bottling this "mineral" water must inject CO_2 back into the water, since it is easily lost between the surface and the bottle. "Seltzer" identifies any water that is carbonated with carbon dioxide; it is often made from filtered tap water. Club soda is essentially the same, though it frequently has more minerals added. All these types of water can also be contaminated, although any bottled carbonated water should be free of microorganisms because they cannot easily live in the presence of carbon dioxide. However, it is important not to drink excessive amounts of carbonated water because the carbon dioxide can affect the body's acid-alkaline balance.

Filtered Water

Home Filters

A good-quality water filter will remove much of the bacterial and chemical contamination from your water. About 2 million home filtering systems are purchased in the United States each year. Filtration, or purification, involves the removal of extraneous matter from water, including bacteria, chemicals, and metals. Legally, anything called a "purifier" must remove 99.75 percent of incoming bacteria. Water can be filtered using a number of methods and medias, including carbon filters, multifilter units (reverse osmosis), and units that make the water more alkaline. Some models fit directly on the faucet and are designed for storage on the countertop or under the sink. Others are available in pitcher styles.

Filtration units are also available that provide filtered water for the entire home. These filters process all the water as it enters the home—not just drinking water, but also water used in showering and washing dishes and clothes. It turns out that we can get a lot of toxins and exposure from the shower that we usually don't think about. The use of more complete filtration removes the toxins in water that are absorbed through the skin during a shower or bath. Although smaller filter units are also available specifically for use in the shower, a good whole-house filter ensures you protection against waterborne toxins and microbes anywhere in the home, because it treats the water at its source.

Carbon Filters

Carbon is the most widely used type of filter. Used for centuries as a filtering substance, carbon provides an extensive porous surface that can absorb contaminants. *Activated carbon* filtration units filter the water mechanically and biomagnetically (ionically) and remove unpleasant coloring, odor, and taste by cleaning the water of bacteria, parasites, most viruses, chlorine, and heavier minerals and matter. Carbon is best at removing organic chemicals and chlorine. The size of the filter determines the types of contaminants it will remove. Basically, a filtration unit should filter out any particles or organisms over 4 microns, which includes most bacteria and parasites, although not viruses.

Carbon is excellent at trapping the larger molecules, chemicals, and larger microorganisms; it is not good at removing inorganic minerals such as the fluoride typically found in municipal waters. However, solid-carbon filtration is believed to be relatively effective at removing many of the toxic minerals with higher molecular weights, such as lead or mercury. The two main types of carbon filters are granulated-carbon filters and solid-carbon block filters.

Granulated-Carbon Filters

Granulated carbon is used in many of the pitcher-style filters and some faucets. There are two primary concerns with these units—the potential for the buildup of bacteria and incomplete filtration. Granulated-carbon filters have air spaces between the carbon particles to trap bacteria and remove them from the water. However, bacteria can multiply within the air spaces. Silver is used in most granulated filters to aid in killing the bacteria. These "silver-impregnated" filters do help to reduce the bacterial growth, but there are still concerns about the gradual accumulation of bacteria and about silver toxicity. Since their use is short-lived, they are not ideal for home use. However, they are often the most convenient for travel. They will remove some chemicals, but our greatest concern is microorganisms. The pore size of the filter is the crucial factor in determining the germs that can be removed. Be sure to check the product information carefully. Table 5.2 shows the sizes of harmful microscopic organisms, measured in microns. *Be sure to use a unit that filters absolutely to 1 micron or finer.*

The pore size of filters varies widely, ranging from 0.5 (the Wellness Water Filter) and 0.2 (the Katadyn unit) to much larger size pores. Portable travel units and pitcher-style filters that have a pore size above 1 micron may not remove parasites such as cryptosporidium.

Solid-Carbon Block Filters

This kind of filtration provides a good basic system that eliminates most microorganism contamination. Since there is very little oxygen within the filtering material, germs are less likely to accumulate. Research has demonstrated that these units also trap more chemicals, organic pollutants, radon, and asbestos than the looser granulated-carbon filters.

Table 5.2 Size of Common Microbes

Microbes	Size (in microns*)
Amoebas	10–50
Giardia lamblia	10–20
Cryptosporidium	2–5
Campylobacter bacteria	0.2–0.3
Cytomegalovirus and herpesvirus	0.15–0.2
HIV	0.1–0.12
Hepatitis viruses	0.025–0.04

*A micron is about 1 millionth of half an inch, or 1 millionth of a centimeter.

Source: Data from J. Nicklin, and others. *Instant Notes in Microbiology.* Oxford: BiosScientific Publishers, 2001.

The filtering surface area of this denser carbon bed can clean more water than granular-carbon filters, and the filters are rated by the volume of water treated. They typically clean 400 to 1000 gallons over the life of the filter, depending on the size of the unit and the amount of sediment in the incoming water. For the most effective filtration, units should be changed once they reach about 75 percent of maximum capacity, to avoid the buildup of bacteria, chemicals, and sediment. Activated carbon filters are usually less expensive than reverse osmosis units.

Reverse Osmosis (RO) Filters

RO filters are also considered a good choice. These systems usually have three different filters and provide extremely thorough filtration. They are thought by some to be the best way to purify water. However, they tend to be more expensive and require good water pressure. Another primary concern with these units is that they may remove too many of the essential trace minerals from the water.

Reverse osmosis units range from small home units to those of industrial size. In this method, tap water flows through special membranes with microporous holes the size of water molecules. These pores allow the water to pass through while trapping the larger molecules of organic and inorganic materials. Reverse osmosis filtration is highly recommended when there is excessive lead in the water because it tends to remove almost all heavy metals. It also removes chemicals such as chlorine, and is one of the few methods that removes fluoride.

These units usually have two or three filtering mechanisms. The first is a sedimentation filter, which allows particles to settle. Second is the reverse osmosis filter, followed by a carbon filter, which removes most of the contaminants that may have passed through the previous membrane. With this system, virtually 100 percent of the organic material is removed, along with almost all minerals. For this reason, there is concern that drinking water devoid of minerals may affect the body's mineral balance and electrolyte activity. This issue needs to be better researched, particularly if the filtration unit provides your primary source of drinking water.

Distilled Water

The distillation process involves vaporizing water (turning it into steam) in one chamber and then condensing it once again into liquid in a separate chamber. This removes the minerals, chemicals, and microbes from the water. Theoretically, distilled water should be pure. However, there is some concern that certain volatile organic chemicals will vaporize and recondense into the second chamber, in the water. For thorough purification, distillation is preceded by solid-carbon filtration.

Distilled water is not recommended for daily usage because this process (like the reverse osmosis process) removes all the minerals from the water. Practitioners report a possible link between long-term use of distilled water and mineral deficiencies. Distilled water may be recommended for use during brief periods of detoxification, due to its ability to draw harmful toxins out of the body. However, there is real concern that over time, use of distilled water may also leach essential minerals out of the body. Recent reports also suggest the risk of higher levels of heavy metals in water that has been distilled.

If you elect to use water filtration, be sure to obtain background information on products before you make a purchase. (Also, see Table 5.3 for tips in minimizing toxins in your water.) Recent research found that some of the most popular filters on

Table 5.3   Minimizing Toxins in Your Water

Type of water or filter	Advantages	Disadvantages
Tap water To check the quality of your tap water, call your water district; useful information on the web can be obtained from www.ewg.org	Inexpensive and available; boil 15 to 20 minutes to remove chlorine, bacteria, and some parasites, especially if you are immune-compromised	Quality varies; often contains chlorine and fluoride; may also contain heavy metals, THMs (trihalomethanes); can contain cryptosporidium, giardia, and other parasites and their cysts
Bottled water Check the label; when ordering bottled water delivery, request testing information; inquire about the source of the water —natural spring, distilled, or filtered municipal water	Usually tested and prefiltered; springwater can be a good natural source of minerals	Soft- and even hard-plastic containers give off toxic gas compounds including plasticizers (phthalates), vinyl chloride, and bisphenol-A (an endocrine disrupter); glass containers are still best
Ceramic carbon filters Two-step filtration with compacted activated carbon and porous ceramic filters	Remove most bacteria, parasites, and cysts; chemicals such as chlorine, pesticides, and most solvents; some radioactive pollutants some heavy metals sediment	These filters do not remove fluoride or certain heavy metals, viruses, or other very small microbes

Table 5.3 *(continued)*

Type of water or filter	Advantages	Disadvantages
Solid-carbon block filters		
With activated carbon; check manufacturer's specifications	Remove chlorine, pesticides, and solvents; some radioactive contaminants	Do not filter out bacteria, asbestos, fluoride, heavy metals, or certain radioactive compounds
Mechanical filters		
Some are impregnated with silver compounds, which destroy bacteria and other microbes	Filter out debris, bacteria, large parasites, and cysts down to 1 or 0.5 microns; also kills some bacteria	Do not filter out asbestos chlorine, fluoride, heavy metals, or THMs, nor most volatile chemicals such as solvents or pesticides
Reverse osmosis filters		
Exceptionally thorough, multistage water filtration that includes membrane and carbon filters	Remove almost everything, except pesticides, radon, and volatile organic chemicals; to compensate, many systems come with add-on carbon filtration units. The two in combination provide the most thorough filtration available	Also remove good minerals and make water "lifeless"; may be supplemented with a unit to add minerals back in; require periodic filter change or back-flushing with chlorine; can outgas plastic compounds into water, requiring an additional filtration step
Granulated-carbon filters, with activated charcoal		
Typically used in small pitcher-style filters, faucet filters, and in some prefilters	Better than drinking unfiltered water; remove some chemicals and particulates, including chlorine, mercury, THMs and larger parasites	Do not filter out bacteria or protozoa under 4 microns in size; nor asbestos, fluoride, certain heavy metals, or most radioactive compounds

Table 5.3 *(continued)*

Type of water or filter	Advantages	Disadvantages
Alkaline water units		
With granulated activated charcoal prefilter (impregnated with silver); can be used in conjunction with carbon block unit for additional filtration	May restore normal acid-base balance in the body and aid detoxification	Same limitations as other granulated charcoal filters; best in combination with prefilter; misses chemicals, fluoride, heavy metals, and viruses

SOURCE: Courtesy Jeffrey Anderson M.D. From What about water? Len Saputo, MD, and Nancy Faass, eds., *Boosting Immunity.* Novato, CA: New World Library, 2002.

the market actually increased the levels of lead in the water, as a result of design flaws within the systems. In addition, some filters have been found to harbor bacteria and then release them into the water. Note that the maintenance of filter systems and regular filter changes are important to assure safe drinking water. (See Resources section at the back of the book.)

Safe Water Tips

1. Avoid tap water as your primary source of drinking water.
2. Minimize your intake of chlorinated and fluoridated water.
3. Determine the most reliable and appropriate type of drinking water for you and your family.
4. Have your regular drinking water assessed to find out your risks.
5. Filter your city or well water.

6. Avoid using tap water in infant's and young children's formula and foods. Never use hot tap water, which can release additional lead and bacteria.
7. When traveling, be extra careful about contaminated water. Boiling it for 15 to 20 minutes will destroy most germs. Or you can use iodine tablets or an appropriate filtration system.
8. Become well informed about drinking water issues.

6

Keeping House

Surface Germs

Fact

A full 80 percent of your germ exposure is to germs you touch.

Germs

Staph, strep, *E. coli*, and other bacteria that originate in the digestive tract, and various molds.

The surfaces in our environment act as intermediaries in the transmission of germs. It has been suggested that 80 percent of the germs we're exposed to are picked up on our hands. So when you are thinking of transmission on surfaces, think in terms of both hands and the surfaces you touch. Simple hygiene such as hand washing and disinfection can reduce the number of germs to a level that your immune system can handle.

Cleaning the House

Let's consider the cleaning of floors and rugs and then look at some of the best approaches to cleaning the rest of the house. A major point to bear in mind is the difference between hard and soft surfaces—hard surfaces include hardwood floors and plastic, wood, and metal, compared with the soft surfaces of rugs, curtains, and fabric. We know that bacteria adhere to both types of surfaces, but researchers have found the bacterial counts on soft surfaces are generally much higher.

Most of us sense that rugs hold a great deal more dust and germs than hardwood floors. The research bears this out. A study conducted by the Municipal Health Service of Amsterdam found that carpeted floors had four times the level of dust as floors with smooth surfaces.[1] Mattresses were also a significant source of mold, as were damp areas in the bedroom. However, the major factor related to the presence of mold was the type of flooring—hard or carpeted. Another study, this one by the Department of Medicine at Northwestern University in Chicago, also compared carpeted and noncarpeted floors, tracking the levels of a particularly nasty bacteria, *Clostridium difficile*. Researchers found that "carpeted floors were significantly more contaminated for prolonged periods with clinical strains of *C. difficile* than were noncarpeted floors."[2]

Dust and molds are unattractive, but they're also major health hazards.

- Indoor mold has been found to have an adverse effect on adult asthma, confirmed in a large European study.[3]
- Some molds are highly toxic, such as aspergillus.[4]

Dust can harbor an entire miniature ecosystem of mold and insects, including dust mites, "volatile organic compounds," carbon dioxide, bacteria, viruses, skin scales, and pet dander. Since levels of dust mites tend to reflect levels of bacteria and mold, this is an important marker of overall cleanliness. Water is another essential ingredient in this ecosystem, water from human sweat, moisture condensed from the air, or water from leaking pipes or walls. "The mixture of moisture and dust, whether . . . in a pillow, a couch, . . . [or] a damp basement . . . will most likely result in the development of a miniature eco-system . . . even on a bathroom ceiling or a basement wall."[5] Maintaining low levels of dust and humidity are the two most important means of avoiding airborne problems and associated health symptoms. Dust mites, which thrive in dust, are a major culprit in triggering asthma.

What are the environmental risk factors for asthma and chronic allergies? The research indicates:

- Location in damp geographic areas associated with increased levels of mold.
- Rugs that had been steam-cleaned.
- No dehumidifier.
- Mold exposure, particularly indoor mold exposure. These exposures were highest in older houses with recent water damage.
- Furred or feathered indoor pets.
- Carpets in the living room.
- Less frequent vacuuming and dusting.

Strategies that reduce the level of dust mites in the environment include:

- Using impermeable or semipermeable covers on mattresses and pillows.
- Eliminating upholstered furniture, carpets, and scatter rugs, at least in the room of the person with asthma. Note that in a study that tracked the effectiveness of rug cleaning in eliminating dust mites, the researchers found that within 3 months, no effect of cleaning could be discerned.[6]
- Washing bed linen with hot water.
- Airing the room daily.
- Minimizing exposure to tobacco smoke.

When there are allergies or asthma in the house, what is the greatest source of allergens? What matters most? A study of 98 Dutch children with asthma sampled the levels of dust in their classrooms, living room and bedroom floors, and mattresses, and tracked other factors in their lives as well.[7] Researchers concluded that carpeted classroom floors did not contribute to the severity of asthma symptoms. The most significant factor found in this study was mattress dust. One effective means of controlling mattress dust is to cover the mattress with an impermeable surface such as a plastic mattress cover or plastic sheeting that can be sealed. Allow the plastic to air out—offgas—sufficiently before using it.

Cleaning Methods

Vacuuming

For anyone with asthma, it can be beneficial to use a high-efficiency vacuum cleaner—a HEPA-type vacuum that will sweep up and retain more of the dust and other particles. The filters in these vacuums are exceptionally fine. In general, vacuums, by the nature of their design, stir up some of the air around them and also recirculate some of the air sucked in by the vacuum. The HEPA-type vacuum retains a greater proportion of the dust it collects because the filter is so fine. As a result, it causes less recirculation of dust and allergens. You can also make your vacuum more efficient by changing the filter more often.

Cleaning and Disinfecting

We know we want a clean house. But what is the best way to accomplish that? When do we need to bring in the heavy-duty cleaners, and when can we use a more natural approach with just soap and water? Cleaning with soap and water is often sufficient to remove any dirt and most of the germs. In other situations, it's important to disinfect—to remove as many germs as possible.

Use of a disinfectant such as household bleach destroys more of the bacteria and other germs. We now know that bacteria, for example, can live on surfaces for up to 2 months. It's especially important to disinfect:

- When there is potential exposure to a high concentration of bacteria
- If someone in the home has been ill, to avoid the possible spread of bacteria

The kitchen is the most potentially dangerous area of the house due to the possibility of infectious bacteria in raw foods, particularly chicken, meat, fish, and eggs. When the person doing the cooking handles these raw foods, those germs can be spread to any other surface he or she touches, including other foods that will not be cooked, such as salads. (See Chapter 4 for more information on kitchen cleanliness.)

Where are the hot spots in your kitchen? Researchers from the University of Arizona ranked objects in a typical kitchen to identify the greatest sources of germs:[8]

- Kitchen sponges and dish cloths were the worst—one sponge can contain more than 6000 bacteria in a square centimeter—more than a million germs on a single sponge.
- The kitchen sink was second, perhaps because meat and poultry are washed there, leaving residues.
- The sink tap handle came in third.
- The refrigerator door was fourth.

A study conducted by the University Hospital of Oslo, Norway, compared four cleaning methods: dry mop, damp mop, wet mop, and wet washing without a mop.[9]

- Dry mopping reduced bacterial levels by 55 percent, although it caused a slight increase in the level of airborne particles. (But another study found that if the dry mop was not cleaned frequently, it could harbor staph bacteria and actually spread them in the process of cleaning.)
- Damp mopping reduced the bacteria counts from the floor by 75 percent.
- Wet mopping had no effect.
- Wet washing without a mop actually increased the level of bacteria on the floor by 35 percent or more!

Although the wet methods didn't always remove germs, they were most effective in removing actual dirt and debris (organic materials) from the floor, by 65 percent or more. Researchers concluded that a combined use of damp mopping and wet mopping is recommended. Another study of cleaning methods found that disposable dust-attracting dry mops retained 59 percent of the bacteria 7 days later. After 2 weeks, the mop still contained more than a fourth of the bacteria.[10] In sum, mops and sponges need to be cleaned or replaced frequently.

Which Disinfectants Work Best?

The research is unanimous about the cleaning ability of bleach. Ammonia was found highly effective in some studies, but in others did not match the cleaning ability of bleach. In the University Hospitals of Geneva, various cleaning methods and disinfectants were compared over a period of 4 months,[11] finding that:

- Bleach was the most effective in reducing the amounts of bacteria.
- Ammonia did not reduce bacteria at all in bathroom and toilet cleaning, but was effective for cleaning furniture. Note that in another study, ammonia was found to effectively reduce the bacteria studied.[12]
- When soap or detergent and water was used, it actually seeded the surfaces with bacteria, increasing their levels.[13]

Use Cleaners with Caution

Cleaners can be hazardous to your health. One case in the medical literature reported on a patient who received chemical burns from a Lysol cleaner and then suffered respiratory distress because he inhaled the fumes. His condition was so severe, it required that he be hospitalized and stay on ventilator support for 3 months.[14]

Safe, Thorough Cleaning

The majority of exposure to cleaners occurs through the skin rather than by inhaling fumes. Toxins can be absorbed through the skin without our awareness. So be sure to wear gloves when you clean. Also wear gloves whenever you clean up body fluids such as vomit, feces, or blood. This is especially important if you

For bathrooms, use:

> ¼ cup bleach
> 1 gallon cool water

This is the same as using 1 tablespoon of bleach to a quart of cool water, in case you want to make up a smaller batch.

Use a weaker solution for disinfecting toys, eating utensils, etc.:

> 1 tablespoon bleach to 1 gallon of cool water

If a family member has a serious illness or if there is an incident involving blood or spoiled meat, extra strong disinfection can be provided by using ⅔ cup of bleach per gallon of water. The research found that even powerful bacteria such as *Staph aureus* and salmonella were reliably inactivated by a solution at that concentration.[15]

have cuts or scratches on your hands. It's also essential if a family member has hepatitis B or C, AIDS, or some other blood-borne disease. Take precautions in any case—even the bacteria that cause flu, food poisoning, or digestive upset can be quite nasty.

Clean surfaces with soap/detergent and water to eliminate organic particles and "dirt." The mechanical action of scrubbing is also important, because it removes the film of bacteria that can adhere to surfaces.

After Cleaning, Disinfect the Area If Needed

Apply bleach diluted in water and leave it on for 5 minutes. Wipe the surface with paper towels that can be thrown away (or cloth towels that can be washed in water and bleach). Note that it is vital that you store disinfectants out of the reach of children. Next wash your gloves and then your own hands.[16]

Disinfectants versus Natural Cleaners

Do natural products work? The answer is that they can work effectively as detergents in the first stage of cleaning. However, research shows clearly that as disinfectants, they are not as effective as traditional cleaners like bleach.

A study conducted at the University of North Carolina tracked the effectiveness of seven familiar cleaners, comparing them with vinegar and also baking soda as disinfectants.[17] The researchers found that most of the commercial products were effective disinfectants. Although the vinegar was quite effective against salmonella and pseudomonas, it was not effective against *Staph aureus* or *E. coli*. Baking soda was not highly effective against any of the four bacteria in the test.

Chemical Sensitivity and Household Cleaners: What's Safe?

There are times when it's important to use a cleaner that we know kills germs—a disinfectant. When a member of the household is ill, this could make the difference between getting sick or staying well. Yet what do we do if someone in the home is chemically sensitive?

Research has clearly established that chemical sensitivity has a physical basis. These conditions can involve the liver, nervous system, immune system, or the body's chemistry. Symptoms may include headaches or migraines, chronic fatigue, aching muscles or joints, difficulty with concentration, sore throats, sinus infections, or asthma. It has also been well documented that people with chemical sensitivity tend to develop symptoms when exposed to toxic chemicals, including cleaning agents and solvents.

The issues become more complicated when we try to identify what's safe and what works. Research has found that the natural cleaners tested did not kill most germs. The cleaners that were effective were ammonia, Clorox bleach, ethanol alcohol, and two phenolic compounds. Yet all these products have a history of toxicity. The FDA has ranked cleaners by their toxic effects:

- **Mild toxicity.** Hydrogen peroxide and Lysol (the type made for hospitals, which contains phenolic compounds, rather than the form made with ammonia)
- **Moderate toxicity.** Bleach

- **Severe toxicity.** Products containing peracetic acid or glutaraldhyde

The potential toxicity of household chemicals to sensitive individuals is reflected in the research. Exposure to these cleaners can be caustic to the skin, causing dermatitis. "Inhalation injury" is know to occur from intense exposure to ammonia or chlorine bleach. Among common household disinfectants, ammonia was associated with the highest number of reports of toxicity—more than a thousand articles in the research literature. Ethanol (alcohol) was most often associated with dermatitis.

Currently, the research on natural cleaners is sparse, and the number of effective products appears to be limited. When tested, baking soda had no disinfectant action. Vinegar killed some bacteria, but not others—nor did it kill viruses. Grapefruit seed extract products performed well against a variety of bacteria in one study, with unclear outcomes in others. Another product that looked promising was a hospital-grade cleaner made with natural extracts—but on closer examination, it also contained ammonia. New hydrogen peroxide products have appeared on the market for use in hospitals and dental offices, but they are too recent to have a track record.

Protective strategies? Use the milder cleaners and save disinfectants for essential times and places (vomit, blood, and bathrooms; cutting boards, kitchen sinks, and counters). If latex allergies are not an issue, use gloves and a dust mask (available from any hardware store). Clean drains with salt and boiling water rather than chemicals.

Minimize other exposures when possible—consider the use of a vacuum with a HEPA filter to cut down on dust and dust mite exposure. Consider working with an integrative physician who specializes in environmental medicine. This approach includes individualized protocol to strengthen the liver and the immune system and to reduce overall sensitivity.

Kids and Germs

It's important to keep a child's room thoroughly clean, particularly in areas such as a diaper-changing table. Other objects and areas that can collect bacteria include toys and crib rails (anything on which children put their mouths) and food preparation areas.

Toys can definitely harbor bacteria. A study of bacteria levels on toys at the doctor's office, conducted by a medical school in New Zealand, found that about 14 percent of the hard toys had evidence of bacteria. However, of the soft toys, as many as 90 percent had moderate to heavy bacteria levels.[18] Another study conducted in a general practitioner's office in Edinburgh, Scotland, found soft toys eight times more likely than hard toys to harbor bacteria.[19] These bacteria can persist. A third study found that shigella bacteria, one of the causes of food poisoning, were evident on utensils, toys, and clothes for as long as 5 days later.[20]

Routine cleaning with soap and water, combined with active scrubbing, reduces the number of germs from the surface, just as the friction reduces germs when you wash your hands. Some objects and surfaces require disinfection as well. Disinfection involves soaking or drenching the items for several minutes with a disinfectant in order to destroy the remaining bacteria. Use commercial products that meet the standards of the Environmental Protection Agency for hospital-grade germicides, such as bleach. However, it's important to remember that as effective as bleach is, it does not destroy all microbes. One example is the protozoa cryptosporidium, periodically found in public water system. Cryptosporidium is only destroyed by ammonia or hydrogen peroxide. Again, be sure to wear gloves when you clean with chemical disinfectants.

Sanitizers can be applied in various ways:

- Using a spray bottle, for diaper changing surfaces and toilets.
- Using cloths rinsed in sanitizing solution for food preparation areas, large toys, books, and activity centers.
- Dipping the object into a container filled with the sanitizing solution, for smaller toys.

It is usually best not to rinse off the sanitizer immediately. Leave the solution on for about 5 minutes. Since chlorine evaporates into the air leaving no residue, surfaces sanitized with bleach may be left to air-dry. Other disinfectants must be rinsed off with fresh water.

Household objects such as telephones can be cleaned at least once a month using alcohol and cotton balls. Remember that almost any common household item can carry or transmit germs—particularly items for personal use. For example, cedar shoe trees, used to keep shoes from shrinking and losing their shape, were found to transmit several hundred to several thousand potentially harmful bacteria and bacterial spores.

Germs on Wood, Fabrics, and Plastic

Hospital studies have found that in general, bacteria can survive on common surfaces and fabrics for a single day to as many as 60 or 90 days if they are not removed in routine cleaning.[21] Researchers also found that bacteria can survive on cotton or polyester clothing or fabric, towels, and plastic. Staph bacteria (*Staphylococci aureas*) survived 1 week on cotton fabric and 2 weeks on terry-cloth toweling. Staph and fecal bacteria survived on synthetic fabrics for days to months. In addition, all bacteria tested survived for at least 1 day on the cotton-polyester blend. Researchers pointed out that these fabrics are typically used in clothing worn by hospital staff—scrub suits, lab coats, and street clothes. The clothing can become a "reservoir" for bacteria as health-care workers move from one patient to the next. Transmission can occur simply by the brush of a sleeve. Candida (a common yeast) was also found to survive on surfaces such as glass, stainless steel, cotton fabric, and cotton-polyester blend. Two species of candida tested remained viable for 3 to 14 days on these surfaces.

Cleaning Hardwood Floors

Dust-mop or vacuum regularly. If you use a mop, run it through the washer frequently. If there is illness in the family, be sure to vacuum rather than mop. If anyone in the family has asthma, consider investing in a HEPA vacuum. Clean hardwood floors using a cleaning agent intended for that purpose. Buff to restore the shine. When this is no longer effective, waxing may be necessary. Properly maintained, a hardwood floor should require waxing only once or twice a year.

Rug Maintenance

Vacuum frequently. Vacuum high-traffic areas daily or at least twice a week. Use a vacuum with an active beater or HEPA filter, and change the bags frequently. Avoid inadequate cleaning of rugs, because soapy residues left on the rug will actually cause them to become resoiled more quickly. Remember that rugs were found to harbor bacteria, so your efforts are not just cosmetic.

Mattresses

Mattresses can be another major source of bacteria. Is it possible to clean a mattress adequately? A study at the University of San Paulo measured surface bacteria levels on 52 mattresses, before and after cleaning. Bacteria were identified in half of the more than 1000 lab tests. Of the samples that tested positive, about half the bacteria were from mattresses before cleaning. Surprisingly, about the same number of mattresses were found to be contaminated after cleaning! The study concluded that rather than getting rid of the bacteria, cleaning merely displaces them and moves them around.[22] This is why it's important (as noted earlier) to use a plastic mattress cover. You can also reduce the level of bacteria and allergens by washing linens, bedding, curtains, and other fabrics in the hot cycle of a washing machine. This usually kills most of the germs.

Minimizing the Exposure — and the Work

Another way to keep dirt and bacteria down is to cut down on the amount of dirt and debris that is tracked in from the outside, for example:

- Provide removable mats at each entrance to your home or apartment, both inside and outside. The mats should be laundered, hosed, or vacuumed whenever they become soiled.
- Consider the habit of taking your shoes off at the door, and keep a pair of slippers or shoes near the door that are only worn inside. This cuts down on the amount of dirt that enters the house to an amazing degree.[23]
- Set aside an area that will function as a mudroom, where outdoor clothing, boots, and shoes can be stored.
- Provide a boot-scraper or decorative boot brush near the door for shoe cleaning.
- Minimize the amount of dirt tracked in by pets by keeping them outdoors or indoors the majority of the time.

Keeping a Clean Bathroom

Fact

There are far fewer germs on your toilet seat than on your kitchen sponge.

Germs

Staph and strep; E. coli and other fecal bacteria; even bacteria such as pseudomonas; viruses; and various species of molds.

Overview

Your kitchen actually harbors more germs than your bathroom! When researchers sampled common household hot spots, they found that the toilet seat was the least contagious area of the home. Perhaps this is because most of us are already aware of the importance of cleaning the bathroom. This is still true: One of the main routes of contagious infection is described as oral-fecal transmission. This refers to the transfer of germs that cling to hands and under fingernails after using the toilet. Since an estimated one-third of the population doesn't bother to wash their hands, this becomes a primary way that germs are passed around. As a result, a great many germs are conveyed on money, telephones, and other surfaces—and also transmitted in food.

A survey by the University of Arizona found that the bathroom and kitchen sinks are among the dirtiest places in the home. These areas call for more thorough cleaning— disinfection—a legal term that means killing harmful bacteria and viruses. In this study, bleach was found to be an effective disinfectant.[24]

You want to have a practical routine that's easy to keep up with. In order to get rid of germs, frequent cleaning is important too. Often the germs are back within 3 to 6 hours, according to a British study.[25] Here are recommendations from the microbiologists at the University of Arizona on keeping ahead of the germs:

- Daily, wipe down sinks and countertops with a cleanser containing chlorine bleach. For example, this will knock out 99.9 percent of fecal organisms.
- Clean faucet handles and other surfaces two or three times a week.
- Do toilets, tubs, and showers once a week. Clean the toilet bowl by adding 1 cup of bleach and letting it stand for 10 minutes or using bleach tablets and then brushing the bowl clean.

You can spot-clean with rubbing alcohol, hydrogen peroxide, or a bleach and water solution in a spray bottle, using tissue or paper towels. You'll also want to use disposables to wipe up spills, since sponges are notorious havens for germs. You can use rubbing alcohol on mirrors, with a paper towel. However, don't put paper towels in the toilet.

Each week, before you scrub the bathroom, vacuum all surfaces to pick up hair and lint.

Other Good Habits

- Close the lid on the toilet before flushing. Avoid the spread of germs which cling to water droplets— aerosol transmission. Microbes tend to float around the bathroom for at least 2 hours if the seat is left open, so you'll want to store your toothbrush in the medicine cabinet, out of harm's way.
- Avoid sharing towels since bacteria and even fungus that cause skin conditions such as tinea can be transmitted on the cloth. This is especially important when a family member is ill—use paper towels instead. Consider putting a paper towel holder in the bathroom.

Making Your Home Less Hospitable to Germs and Mold

Most microbes thrive in damp environments. Keep the bathroom dry and well ventilated to reduce the levels of bacteria and mold. A humidity level below 40 percent will definitely discourage mold. You can keep the humidity down by using a strong dehumidifier, but remember to keep it clean and disinfected as well. Mold inhibitors can be added to bathroom paint. Do not carpet bathrooms since carpets and rugs hold moisture, creating the ideal environment for mold (and bacteria) to thrive. Bleach is known to be a particularly good antifungal.

Rubbing alcohol (isopropyl alcohol in a 70 percent solution) that you can purchase at any drugstore seems to be effective against mold and bacteria, particularly for spot cleaning. In order to be effective, leave it on the surface for 5 to 10 minutes. It will evaporate and leave no odor.

Specifics

- **Sinks.** If you are living in your own home, you may want to replace old sinks that have pitted surfaces. Abraded sinks retain more germs, according to research, and stainless steel sinks tend to collect less bacteria. "Surfaces with poor cleanability . . . were characterized by pitting, crevices, or jags." These surfaces are likely to retain more bacteria because of increased numbers of attachment sites.[26]
- **Drains.** Keep drains clean. They've been found to harbor nasty microbes.
- **Soaps.** Several types of bacteria can survive on bar soap, so liquid soap is a safer approach—particularly if there are a number of people in the household sharing the soap.
- **Sponges.** The structure of a sponge is an ideal environment for bacteria and molds—dark, moist, with innumerable hiding places. We know now that sponges are the worst source of germs. A number of studies also found that when we clean with a contaminated sponge or cloth, we either move the germs around or increase their numbers, making our home more germ-infested than if we hadn't cleaned at all![27]

- **Shower sponges.** Shower sponges are also highly subject to bacteria. Our skin sheds about 1.5 million flakes every hour, along with the *Staph aureus* bacteria that normally occurs on skin. "In an environment as humid as the bathroom, a single bacteria cell can multiply into one billion clones overnight."[28]
- **Toothbrushes.** Toothbrushes should never be placed wet in the case, due to the potential for mold or possibly bacteria. However, they should not be left out in the room, with the potential for contamination by bacteria in spray from the toilet.
- **Mouthwash.** Use a disposable cup since germs can be left on the rim of the bottle whenever anyone takes a sip directly.
- **Towels.** Bacteria and even viruses survive on towels through every stage of laundering, especially when they're washed in warm or cold water. Here are steps to minimize problems:
  - Wash underwear separately in hot water (at least 155°F).
  - Add bleach or a detergent with a sanitizer to all wash loads containing underwear.
  - Disinfect the machine, if you need to, by running an empty cycle with bleach and water.
  - Line-dry your clothes in the sun if you have this option, so that the ultraviolet rays can kill the germs.[29]

7

Airborne Germs
and Molds

Airborne Molds and Mold Spores

Fact

The beautiful sunsets of south Florida are caused by African
dust storms that originate in the Sahara Desert. The dust
plumes are carried on the wind and reach the Caribbean and
the Americas in about 5 to 7 days. High levels of microbes were
found in one test to correlate with weather mapping of the dust
storms. Airborne dust has been identified as the primary source
of allergic stress worldwide.

Germs

Molds, mildew, and other fungi are common pollutants often
found inside the house. In the warmest areas of the United
States, especially those with high humidity, molds thrive year-
round. Indoor molds can flourish even in the coldest climates
and cause allergy symptoms. They tend to occur in areas where
humidity levels are high, such as is the case in bathrooms,

kitchens, laundry rooms, and basements. Mold spores can cause fungal infections that can be quite serious in immune-compromised people, including mold species such as:

- **Aspergillus species.** Fungal spores inhaled from organic matter, such as leaves in the forest
- **Histoplasmosis.** Fungal spores in the old droppings of birds or bats
- **Coccidioides.** Spores in the air-blown dust from desert regions where this fungus grows in the soil. This species can cause respiratory infections and in some cases systemic infection with more generalized effects.

In terms of allergies and asthma, of all airborne micro-organisms, fungi are the greatest concern.

Overview

There are thousands of types of yeasts and mold, two groups in the fungus family. Yeasts are single cells that divide to form clusters. Molds consist of multiple cells that grow as branching filaments or thread-like structures. Unlike plants, they are unable to produce their own food from sunlight and air. Instead, they must live on plant or animal matter, which they slowly break down for their nourishment. Dust mites and animal dander are often associated with airborne molds and microbes, because they tend to accumulate in the environments that promote molds and bacterial growth.

Fungi can live on even minimal amounts of organic matter found in any household. A great many of the fungal species can survive on the structural materials found in the average home, including wood, carpet, carpet backing, cloth, and paper. Fungi are also able to survive in air distribution systems, air filters, and insulation within these systems. Even moderate disturbances in air flow, such as walking on a carpet, sitting on a couch, or vacuuming, can dislodge spores and make them airborne. That said, it's encouraging to know that good hygiene and maintenance of a streamlined environment will tend to minimize mold in most homes.

It's important to be aware that mold can pose a serious threat to human health. Chronic water leaks, standing water, or water saturation of the walls or structure of a residence can support the growth of large quantities of molds and mold spores. These situations require the evaluation of a professional who is knowledgeable in this area.

Common Sources of Mold

- **Paper and fabrics.** Some molds grow on materials such as books and paper, curtains, upholstered furniture, and carpeting.
- **Food sources.** Mold can grow on various foods and on grease, dirt, and soap scum.
- **Wood and soil.** Certain types of mold thrive in wood and soil, so they may grow in the soil of potted plants, on unfinished wooden surfaces, and on papers and newspapers. If you have a fireplace, this is one of the reasons not to store the wood inside.
- **Mattresses.** Your mattress can be one of the worst sources of molds, bacteria, and viruses (according to research), so you'll want to encase it in a nonporous plastic covering. Avoid foam

rubber pillows and mattresses. Replace your pillows frequently.

- **Refrigerators.** Mold tends to grow around door gaskets.
- **Laundry.** Dry clothing immediately after washing, and vent the clothes dryer to the outdoors to keep the humidity level and lint out of your home.
- **Garbage cans.** Empty these containers frequently and disinfect them periodically to prevent the growth of mold.
- **Bathrooms.** As we all know, mold also tends to adhere to surfaces such as the grout between the tiles in the bathroom. Open the window or use an exhaust fan in the bathroom to remove humidity after showering. Use a squeegee to remove excess water from the shower stall, tub, and tiles. This is a better option than a sponge or cloth, which can easily harbor microbes and actually increase the level of bacteria on surfaces. Don't carpet your bathroom. If you use a mat, wash it weekly and include bleach in the wash.
- **Closets.** Since closets typically have poor ventilation, they may be prone to mold, particularly if they are damp. For this reason, dry your shoes, boots, and raincoats thoroughly before storing.
- **Basements.** Molds often flourish in dark, damp places where water pools, such as basements. Thus, it's important not to locate bedrooms on the basement level of a house. Cinder-block or brick walls can be coated with a paint that contains a mold inhibitor. Carpets and padding should not be

laid on a concrete floor. Vinyl flooring is a better choice.
- **Crawl spaces.** A dirt subbasement area or dirt floor can be covered with plastic, which will serve as a vapor barrier to some degree.
- **Almost anywhere!** Moisture and warmth can accelerate the growth of dormant mildew spores on most surfaces.

The Effects of Molds

Many molds and mildews reproduce by generating spores. The spores can float throughout the house, forming new colonies when they land on substances and environments that support their growth. The airborne mold spores, when inhaled, can produce allergy symptoms, so you'll want to take mold seriously. Be aware that a mold colony just 4 inches in diameter can produce millions of spores—enough to cause an allergic reaction or even an asthmatic attack in a sensitive person or a young child. Some molds generate toxins, so they're referred to as "toxigenic." Familiar molds include stachybotrys and aspergillus.

Symptoms linked to mold infestations and also "sick building syndrome" can include:

- Respiratory problems—runny nose, sneezing, nasal congestion, coughing, or difficulty breathing
- Sinus congestion or chronic serious infection
- Allergies and asthma (dust mites have been identified as the single most important trigger for asthma)
- Headaches

- Dizziness or difficulty with concentration
- Fatigue—in some cases, chronic fatigue

Caution: Toxigenic fungi tend to cause acute symptoms only when there is massive building contamination. *Stachybotrys atra* is one of the most toxigenic species of mold. It grows on wood or paper that has been exposed to water for long periods of time. Exposure to stachybotrys can occur through ingestion, contact with contaminated materials, or inhalation of airborne spores. Symptoms include diarrhea, headache, and extreme fatigue, and in young infants this fungus can cause fatal bleeding in the lungs.

Identifying Mold

In some situations, you can see or smell mold colonies growing on surfaces. For example, mold on foods and in bathrooms is visible. And mold in books and mildew on clothing can often be smelled.

Suspect mold growth wherever there are water stains, standing water, or moist surfaces. Damp basements or crawl spaces are notorious havens for mold growth.

In addition, remember that mold is surprisingly adaptable and takes many forms. For example, it may simply look like the soot from car exhaust that gathers on aluminum window frames and on window glass.

Basic testing is available that can be performed at home and sent to a lab. You can find more information about testing later in the chapter and at the back of the book in the Resources section.

Preventing or Clearing Mold

Mold growth can be minimized by keeping basements, bath-rooms, and other rooms clean and dry:

- **Disinfectants.** Use a disinfectant to clean surfaces that have mold on them.
- **Cleaning and sealing wood.** Bare wood can be cleaned with a 50 percent bleach solution, left on for 24 hours. Wood surfaces should be sanded and well sealed with several coats of a hard-finish polyurethane or varnish.
- **Carpeting or furnishings.** When carpeting or furnishings become wet, they must be thoroughly dried as quickly as possible and cleaned or else discarded.
- **Low humidity.** Keep humidity below 50 percent— ideally between 35 and 40 percent—by making sure there is good ventilation and by using a dehumidifier when necessary. (Some units are quieter than others, so whenever possible, check out a floor model before you purchase your unit.) Gauges are available from building supply stores to monitor the humidity level. Avoid overhumidi-fication in the winter.
- **Carpeting.** Those who are sensitive may find it helpful to replace carpeting with hard surfaced flooring and use area rugs that can be removed and cleaned. (See Chapter 6 for more suggestions on cleaning the surface in your home.)

- **Vacuums with high-efficiency HEPA filters.** These can help to reduce airborne dust that is recirculated in the process of vacuuming.
- **Air conditioners and vent openings.** If the source of the mold is outside the home, the most effective way to eliminate it is to filter it out before it enters the house by using a window unit. The filters in air conditioners and vent openings can be used to trap molds at the point of entry.
- **Freestanding air filters.** To minimize molds within the home, a freestanding air cleaner or "air scrubber" can be effective. It is important to get a good-quality unit, such as those manufactured by Austin. Vents and central furnace filters can also be helpful in removing airborne mold.
- **Humidifiers, dehumidifiers, and air conditioning units.** Be sure to be clean these appliances regularly with a disinfectant such as chlorine bleach.
- **Convection heat units.** Since these units warm the air and reduce the humidity, they can reduce the spread of mold and mildew.
- **Testing.** Mold test kits simply involve taking a sample using a petri dish—a small, flat plastic dish that contains a thin layer of hard gelatin (agar). To take a sample, the lid is removed and the dish is placed face down on the surface to be tested. After an hour, the lid is placed back on the dish. The dish is kept in a room of moderate temperature for about a day to enable the mold to begin growing and then is shipped to the lab for evaluation. Lab reports indicate the type of mold and the number of spores identified,

which provides some sense of whether the mold growth is minor or extreme.

Airborne Viruses and Bacteria

Airborne particles are a major cause of respiratory ailments, with the potential to cause allergies, asthma, and infections.

Fact

A *sneeze*. During a sneeze, millions of tiny droplets of water and mucus are expelled at about 200 miles an hour (more than 300 feet per second!). The droplets are initially about 10 to 100 micrometers in diameter, but they quickly dry to become droplet nuclei of about 1 to 4 micrometers. Droplet nuclei contain virus particles or bacteria. They are a major means of disease transmission in humans.[1]

Germs

Important diseases transmitted from person-to-person as airborne particles include:

- **Viral infections.** Chicken pox, the common cold, flu, German measles, measles, mumps, and smallpox are all caused by viruses. Infections in the nose and throat are often caused by viruses due to "droplet transmission." They typically affect the upper airways, rather than the lungs. Most bacterial diseases are also initiated in the upper airways, carried through droplets or adhered to tiny particles.

- **Bacterial infections.** Diphtheria, bacterial meningitis, pneumonia, and tuberculosis, are all caused by bacteria.

Infectious diseases caused by viruses and bacteria occur through various routes of transmission: from person to person, airborne—for example, the bacteria that cause whooping cough (pertussis) and *H. influenzae*, which can cause pneumonia or meningitis. Others are conveyed in the environment, such as psittacosis from dried droppings of infected pigeons, parrots, or other birds.

In addition, certain bacteria are highly adapted to a particular environmental niche. Legionnaires' disease is spread by droplets from air-conditioning systems or water storage tanks where the bacteria grow. Originally legionella, the bacterium that causes Legionnaires' disease, was simply soil bacteria before it adapted to an existence within buildings' ventilation systems.

Airborne particles also cause:

- **Allergies.** There tends to be less knowledge about bacteria as a trigger of allergies, with symptoms that resemble head colds or even asthma. When microorganisms are the source of the allergy, they can cause sensitivity even if the bacteria are no longer alive. This means that in order to minimize allergies, once the bacteria are killed with a disinfectant, they still must be removed mechanically by thorough cleaning such as scrubbing or vacuuming.

- **The common cold.** This familiar infectious illness,
  which affects the upper respiratory tract, can be
  caused by any of more than 100 types of viruses. There
  is currently no known cure and no preventive drug,
  although in our experience the use of certain key
  nutritional supplements can frequently prevent or
  shorten the course of the illness.
- **Tuberculosis.** Unlike typical viruses and bacteria,
  more serious airborne infections such as tuberculosis
  tend to be initiated deep in the lungs. Tuberculosis
  is typically acquired through close contact with a
  diseased person.
- **Emphysema and chronic bronchitis.** These
  conditions are now found to be triggered by infections
  from new strains of common germs. In some cases,
  the infections have been linked to more serious
  illness, such as chronic obstructive pulmonary disease,
  the fourth-leading cause of death in the United States.
  The new microbe strains most often implicated
  include strep bacteria and *H. influenzae*. Since
  H. influenzae is normally found in the throat of about
  75 percent of healthy adults and children, this is
  another reminder of the importance of having strong
  immunity.
- **Hypersensitivity to toxins.** Some airborne microbes
  produce toxins that can affect the quality of indoor air.
  Bacteria are known to produce endotoxins, blamed for
  symptoms associated with hypersensitivities.

Prevention

Strategies for avoiding airborne microorganisms include:

- Minimizing dust, bacteria, and molds in your home
- Identifying and eliminating as many allergies as possible to keep your respiratory tract healthy
- Avoiding colds and flu, or addressing them at the first sign
- Minimizing exposure to respiratory toxins and contagion whenever possible.

8

Kids and Germs

How Germs Are Spread
from Person to Person

Illnesses that are transmitted from person to person are described as contagious or communicable.

Basically, in order for germs to be spread from one person
to another, three things must happen:

1. Germs must be present in the environment. The
    source may be:
    - A person carrying the germs
    - Body fluids or wastes that are infectious, such as
      stool, or semen or discharge from the eyes, nose,
      or mouth
    - Bacteria or viruses in the air
    - Germs on surfaces or objects

2. A person who hasn't yet been exposed to the germ
    must come in contact with it—or he or she may have
    been exposed, but hasn't yet developed immunity to
    that particular germ.

3. The contact or exposure must happen in a way that leads to infection.

Germs often survive by transmission from one person to another. In other cases, they may be conveyed from people to animals and then back to people. Transmission can occur through the air we breathe, through food or water we ingest, or through our skin (by direct contact, infected cuts, or insect bites). About 80 percent of all disease transmission occurs through touch (and so hand washing is one of the major ways we can break the cycle). Person-to-person transmission can occur through several primary routes, as discussed in the following sections and summarized in Table 8.1.

Table 8.1   Person-to-Person Transmission of Germs

Direct contact	Respiratory transmission	Fecal-oral transimssion	Blood transmission
Chicken pox*	Chicken pox*	Campylobacter	Cytomegalovirus
Cold sores	Common cold	E. coli	Hepatitis B*
Conjunctivitis	Diphtheria*	Enterovirus	Hepatitis C
Head lice	Fifth disease	Giardia	HIV infection
Impetigo (skin rash)	Hand-food-and-mouth disease	Hand-foot-and-mouth disease	
Ringworm	Impetigo	Hepatitis A*	
Scabies	Influenza*	Infectious diarrhea	
	Measles*	Pinworms	
	Bacterial meningitis*	Polio*	
	Mumps*	Salmonella	
	Pertussis*	Shigella	
	Pneumonia		
	Rubella*		

* Vaccines are available for preventing these diseases.

Source: CDC. How some childhood infectious diseases are spread: Method of transmission. *ABC's of Safe and Healthy Child Care.* Web site: www.cdc.gov/ncidod/hip/abc/intro.htm: page 2. Accessed June 2002.

Direct Contact

Germs can be transmitted through direct contact with an infected person's skin or body fluid. They may be transmitted in body secretions—mucus, saliva, stool, or semen. Someone who is ill can spread the germs in a number of ways:

- By touching, for example, a handshake
- By kissing
- Through contact with fluid from an infected area of the skin, when there is a condition such as chickenpox or an infected cut
- Through contact by touching a surface that carries germs from a cough or sneeze—or that has been touched by the infected person—such as a telephone or money

Respiratory Transmission

In person-to-person transmission that is airborne, germs are conveyed from the lungs, throat, or nose of one person to another. Colds, for example, can be spread when those who are well:

- Inhale the cold virus carried on tiny airborne droplets of moisture (saliva or mucus) from the nose and throat of an infected person, through a cough or sneeze
- Unknowingly have even microscopic droplets of this fluid on their hands and then touch their eyes, mouth, or nose

Germs can also simply be transmitted in the air at close range.

Fecal-Oral Transmission

For parents or caregivers of young children, for example, this type of transmission can result from contact with feces or objects contaminated with feces.

- Diaper changing can involve direct contact with stool. Microscopic bits of matter and germs or parasite cysts can remain lodged under the fingernails and be absorbed when the new host touches his or her eyes or mouth or touches food.
- Many people also pick up a few germs in the normal course of using the toilet. These germs tend to cling to the hands or lodge under the fingernails. Since about one-third of the population doesn't wash their hands, these germs can be transmitted to the surfaces and the people they encounter. When food handlers don't bother to wash their hands, their customers (or their family) are at risk.
- Microbes from stool can also be spread in food. One of the most devastating E. coli outbreaks on record occurred when tiny bits of manure stuck to the surface of freshly picked apples. The apples were juiced, and since the juice was not pasteurized (cooked), the bacteria were not destroyed and remained in the juice.

Blood Transmission

Transmission through blood can occur in conjunction with an accident, in a medical setting through transfusions, or during intravenous drug use from shared needles.

- Blood infections are spread when blood (and sometimes other body fluids) from a person with an infection gets into the bloodstream of an uninfected person. This can occur when infected blood (or body fluid) enters the body of an uninfected person:

- Through cuts or openings in the skin
- Through contact with the mucous membranes that line body cavities such as the nose, rectum, and vagina
- Through direct transmission into the bloodstream, for example, through an injection

Some diseases, such as chicken pox, impetigo, and hand-foot-and-mouth disease, can have more than one route of transmission. For example, they may spread through the air or by direct contact with the infectious germ.

When Someone in the Family Is Ill

The home is one of the places where germs are most often transmitted. When any member of the household becomes ill, he or she can introduce the germs to others, since each member of the family:

- Comes in contact with the same environment
- Breathes the same air and lives in close proximity to the others
- Uses the same bathroom (which is why scrupulous cleaning is so important)
- Touches surfaces and objects that may contain microscopic traces of bacteria or viruses carried by others

Breaking the Cycle at Home

If there is illness in the household, the primary goal is to minimize the spread of germs. The goal is to block transmission—to break the cycle. This usually means adjusting some of your routines.

- **Hand washing is key**. When cooking, wash your hands and the exposed portions of your arms with soap and warm water and then use a nailbrush.

- **Making the bed.** A Japanese study of hospital bed making found that the number of germs in the air was significantly higher 15 minutes after bed making. The bacteria counts returned to normal 30 to 60 minutes later. However, bacteria were found on many surfaces in the room, suggesting that the bacteria were recirculated in the air, while making the bed.[1] When making the bed, carefully gather up the linens to avoid raising a lot of dust and circulating airborne germs. Minimize the airborne transmission of germs when cleaning up after a family member who has been ill and also when disinfecting the room.

- **Going the extra cleaning mile.** If a family member has a serious illness or if there is an incident involving blood or spoiled meat, extra strong disinfection can be provided using bleach at (2½ tablespoons per quart of water or ⅔ cup of bleach to a gallon of water). The research found that even powerful bacteria such as *Staph aureus* and salmonella were reliably inactivated by a solution at that concentration.[2]

- **Using washing machines and dishwashers.** Wash clothing, towels, and bedding separately in hot water. The use of a dishwasher can also be extremely effective in killing germs because it utilizes very hot water.

- **Disinfecting the bathroom.** When there is illness or when your bathroom gets particularly heavy use, here's a more stringent routine:[3]

Daily, quick-clean with a bleach solution, letting it stand and then wipe it clean with paper towels after 30 seconds. Use this method to:
- Spray-clean the sink and countertops.
- Clean the toilet seat, handle, and floor around the toilet.

Three times a week, clean other areas by letting them soak in bleach and water for 10 minutes:
- Fill the sink with water and 1 cup of bleach to soak.
- Add 1 cup of bleach to the toilet.
- Mop the floor with a solution of 1 cup of bleach to each gallon of water.

Weekly:
- Add 1 cup of bleach to the toilet bowl, let it soak for 10 minutes, and then clean it with a brush.
- Spray the surface of the bath or shower with a bleach solution and then rinse after 5 minutes.

Children

Children tend to be especially vulnerable to contagious illness. The youngest have not yet been exposed to most common germs. Since they are only immune to diseases they have already encountered, their immunity is limited. Once they enter school, their exposure is often greater—this is true at any age, from kindergarten to college. Given this increased exposure, what can we do that will make the greatest difference?

Building Your Child's Immunity

There are a number of basic steps you can take to strengthen your child's immunity. You may find it helpful to look over the information on building immunity included throughout the book. The Resources section at the end of the book also suggests additional information that will help you provide your child with a strong foundation for good health.

1. **Minimize sugar.** We know that sugar can decrease white cell function—our vital infection fighters—and impair the efficiency of the immune system. Sugar has also been implicated in dozens of diseases, including heart disease and diabetes. One of the keys is to find healthy snacks that taste good to your child—fresh fruits, nuts, whole-grain crackers, and other wholesome choices.

2. **Limit the intake of trans fats.** These harmful fats, found in deep-fried foods and in margarine, interfere with normal function of the body. Instead, provide essential fats for optimum health.

3. **Eliminate allergy triggers.** This lightens the burden on the immune system. Many children are sensitive to milk or wheat. This sometimes becomes apparent just by avoiding an offending food for a week and then adding it back into the diet to see if an allergic reaction will occur. We now have so many delicious foods to substitute for these products that an allergy-free diet is no longer the challenge it once was.

4. **Provide children with the essential nutrients.** The immune system uses vitamin A and zinc as building blocks to make immune artillery. You can supplement these nutrients by giving cod liver oil and a good multivitamin. You can also support your children's immune function with transfer factors. These are the microscopic blueprints our immune systems relies on

to recognize and combat germs. Transfer factors are found in the colostrum of the mother's first milk. Although colostrum contains less than 1 percent transfer factors, these factors are the most important component of the colostrum. This vital immune support is now available in supplement form, in a product called Transfer Factor.

These steps can be especially important when a young child starts day care. Whenever the body encounters novel germs for the first time, combating them requires additional effort by the immune system. You can strengthen your child against illness by:

- Strengthening the immune function
- Minimizing stress on the immune system

Minimizing Food Poisoning

Given the range of possible conditions that children can contract, what are the illnesses American children experience most often? The Centers for Disease Control tracks the occurrence of disease across the country on a weekly basis. This chapter includes the CDC's data on the most frequent contagious illnesses reported for children in the year 2000, summarized by age group.

Food-borne illness is currently one of the major challenges to the health of our children. For the very young, the primary issue is vulnerability. In infants, toddlers, and preschoolers, the immune system has not yet fully matured. Their digestive tracts are also immature. As a result, young children are one of the age groups most likely to experience food poisoning. The number of reported cases for children ages 1 to 4 is about 15,000 (see

Table 8.2). Generally the CDC estimates the actual number of cases to be much higher. Food poisoning due to salmonella, for instance, may occur about 40 times as often as reported. If this is true, every year more than 1 million very young children suffer from food poisoning.

A look at the data on elementary school–aged children shows almost an equal number of cases at that age. Factors include more meals eaten in fast-food restaurants and school cafeterias and more deli food and prepared meals since about two-thirds of mothers now work. So it is possible that 1 million elementary school–aged children may also contract food poisoning each year.

The potential severity of food poisoning is another reason it merits attention. Among all age groups, 6000 to 9000 fatalities from food poisoning are reported each year. Each case

Table 8.2   Illnesses That Affect Children 1 to 4 Years Old (Year 2000)

From food and water	Number of cases reported
Cryptosporidium infections	670
Hemorrhagic E. coli infections	835
Hepatitis A	721
Salmonella infections	6,443
Shigella infections	6,701
Total	15,370
Insect-borne illness	
Lyme disease	1,020
Airborne illness	
Pertussis (whooping cough)	787
Resistant strep pneumonia	1,176
Tuberculosis	454
Total	2,417

SOURCE: Data from CDC. Summary of Notifiable Diseases—United States, 2000. *Morbidity and Mortality Weekly Report.* 2002, June 14; 49 (53): 1–102.

reflects a personal tragedy. The most unfortunate of these are child fatalities—statistics can never convey the grief and tragedy of the needless death of a child. Each one of those deaths translates into a life held dear, such as Kevin, who died when he was just 2 years old; Tyler, at 3; and Alex, who died when he was 11.

What You Can Do

- Set a good example.
- Be mindful of the choices you and your family are making, whether you're dining out or eating in, both in terms of the foods you serve and your own kitchen hygiene. Involve your children in decision-making, listen to their input, and take them seriously. In addition:
  - Teach them to wash their hands well.
  - Select a day-care situation that is conscientious about food preparation and hand washing.
  - When you dine out with your children, choose restaurants that are clean and reputable. Use fast food selectively, as a treat.
- Practice the safest possible food handling at home:
  - Pack safe lunches for school or day care. (See Chapter 4 for suggestions on packing a safe lunch.)
  - Cook meats, poultry, and eggs thoroughly.
  - Purchase these protein foods from organic sources whenever possible.
  - Learn to enjoy other sources of protein besides meat, such as eggs, cheeses, yogurt, and organic milk, tofu and other soy products, as well as nuts and seeds.

- Don't give young children unpasteurized soft cheeses like Camembert or raw milk.
- Wash all fruits and vegetables thoroughly.

Preschoolers

Fact

At least 5.8 million children under the age of 5 attend some type of child-care center.

About 65 percent of women with children age 5 or younger were part of the labor force in 1998.

Kids and Day Care

The good news is that children who attend day care tend to have fewer illnesses once they get older, according to research.[4] Exposure to a variety of germs can be positive as long as the child doesn't develop illness too frequently. On the other hand, being in day care increases the risk of illness, particularly in very young children who still have immature immune systems and limited immunity. Since they only develop immunity to each specific illness once they are exposed to it, their early years are a kind of training period for the immune system.

Toddlers also tend to get sick more often than older children because they put their fingers and objects in their mouths and because they spend a great deal of time on the floor. In addition, some diseases have more than one route of infection. For example, colds and flu can be transmitted as airborne germs in a cough or a sneeze. The cold virus (hidden in mucus) can also be conveyed by touch, by objects, or even by food. For this reason, it is important to practice good hygiene when your children are young. This means developing simple, practical routines that focus on the things that make the greatest difference, such as safe handling of protein foods and clean bathrooms.

Criteria for Choosing a Child-care Center

When selecting day care for a child, it's important to choose a center that makes hygiene one of its priorities. From this point of view, it can be instructive to look at how the space and routine are managed. The spread of germs can be minimized by avoiding overcrowding, maintaining good ventilation, and keeping the center clean. If you are in the process of selecting a child-care center, you may find it helpful to review the CDC's guidelines for centers and caregivers. The CDC offers these recommendations for early childhood illnesses:

- It's important that all children and adults use good hand washing practices.
- Children should be taught basics such as covering their mouths when they cough and using tissues when they sneeze.
- Toys, tables, chairs, and other surfaces need to be cleaned and disinfected daily.
- Overcrowding should be avoided to minimize the spread of germs. If the children nap too close together, they're more likely to pick up airborne germs from one another.
- Good ventilation must be provided by opening the windows or doors, or by using an effective ventilation system.

A Quick Note on Hand Washing

We've talked a number of times about the importance of hand washing. An interesting study bears this out. Researchers videotaped very young children at home and at day care and then analyzed their movements. They found that the children touched their food on average 19 times during a meal.[5] Their food only touched the table about five times during the meal. Since hands are the major point of contact with food, good hand washing is one of the most positive habits you can encourage.

Day Care and Food

The research on kids, food, and day care contains good news and bad. The bad news is that germs can proliferate in day-care settings, just as they do in any other group environment or institution. Bad bugs found in day-care centers have included cryptosporidium, rotavirus, *E. coli*, and Norwalk virus.

The good news is that the research confirmed the beneficial effects of simple actions parents can take, such as minimizing allergies and providing a healthy diet. If you have a child who is attending day care, you'll also want to become informed about the quality of the food and the food-handling practices. For example, do the employees use safe dish-washing methods? This means use of a dish-washing machine or a three-step process with a bleach rinse.

Diaper Changing

The same germs that cause food poisoning can be transmitted by way of the oral-fecal route in any environment where there are young children in diapers. The oral-fecal route simply means exposure to microscopic particles of stool (and germs) that can be transmitted during diaper changing, potty training, and using the toilet. The cysts of various protozoa are often transmitted by touch, harbored under fingernails or on hands that weren't adequately washed. Changing tables should be cleaned frequently, and workers should wash their hands every time they change diapers and again before preparing food. In fact, if you have a toddler, avoid using the changing tables provided in public places due to the risk of contamination by germs.

Bad Bugs in Day Care

As a result of increased exposure, the spread of bacteria and other microbes in a day-care setting can be surprisingly pervasive. For example, rates of giardia (a microscopic parasite) tend to be high in day-care centers. In a Johns Hopkins study of 31 day-care centers, about 20 percent of the children had giardia.[6] A Denver study found that 16 percent of children in day care had giardia, compared with 9 percent of those cared for at home.[7] A New Hampshire study suggested that attendance in day care increased the risk of giardia by 50 percent.[8] Several of the studies pointed out that some of the children who were infected had no symptoms, and doctors report that this type of infection is often missed in laboratory testing. Antibody testing, called ELISA, tends to be one of the more reliable approaches to detecting the infection. These infections usually respond well to treatment with medication and improved hygiene, once they've been identified.

Cleaning and Disinfection

In order to avoid infections such as giardia, hygiene needs to be a high priority in a day-care environment. Reducing the levels of germs is another way to reduce the burden on the immune system. The surfaces most likely to be contaminated are the areas of frequent contact—toys, crib rails, food preparation areas, and diaper-changing areas. Washing and disinfection are ideally done several times a day—and at least once daily. Good scrubbing with soap and water reduces the level of germs on surfaces. In addition, some items and surfaces should also be disinfected after cleaning with soap and rinsing with clear water. This involves the use of a chemical such as bleach, which is stronger than soap and proven to kill bacteria and viruses. Commercial products that meet the EPA's standards for "hospital-grade" germicides (germ-killing solutions) can be used. For more suggestions, see Chapter 6 on surface germs and cleaning. The Centers for Disease Control provides in-depth information on hygiene in day-care settings, intended for caregivers and parents.

Cleaning Toys

The CDC recommends that infants and toddlers not share toys—this is particularly true of toys in day care or at home when there is illness in the family. In day-care settings, the toys that children put in their mouths need to be washed and disinfected between use by individual children, so the most appropriate toys are those that are washable. One strategy for controlling germs is to retrieve each toy from the playing area once a child has finished playing with it, and put it in a bin reserved for dirty toys, out of reach. The toys can then be washed at a more convenient time later, and transferred to a bin for clean toys where they can be reused by other children without the risk of transmitting a contagious illness. (Remember that illness is most transmittable *before* the symptoms are apparent.)

To wash and disinfect a hard-plastic toy, scrub it in warm, soapy water, using a brush to reach into the crevices. Rinse the toy in clean water and then immerse it in a mild bleach solution (1 tablespoon of bleach to 1 gallon of water) and soak it in the solution for 10 to 20 minutes. Then remove the toy, rinse it, and air-dry it. Stuffed toys are most appropriate for use by a single child and should be cleaned in a washing machine at least once a week or more frequently.

Exclusion Due to Illness

You'll also want to be sure that the center you choose has a clear policy on attendance during illness. The following are the CDC's recommendations on when children should be excluded due to illness:

- Fever and sore throat, rash, vomiting, diarrhea, earache, irritability, or confusion. Fever is defined as having a temperature of 101°F when taken orally, 100°F or higher when taken under the arm, or 102°F when taken rectally. For children 4 months or younger, a lower rectal temperature of 101°F is considered a fever threshold.
- Diarrhea—runny, watery, or bloody stools.
- Vomiting—two or more times in a 24-hour period.
- Body rash with fever.
- Sore throat with fever and swollen glands.
- Severe coughing—child gets red or blue in the face or makes high-pitched whooping sound after coughing.
- Eye discharge—thick mucus or pus draining from the eye or other signs of eye infection.
- Yellowish skin or eyes.

- Irritability, continuous crying, and the need for attention to such a degree that it would impinge on the health and safety of other children in the center.

Kids and Antibiotics

As most parents can tell you, the transmission of germs and infections is definitely amplified in day-care centers and schoolrooms. As a result, antibiotics can become pervasive in our children's lives. One study found that young children attending day care were 36 times more likely to contract serious infections than those who remained at home.[9,10] In 1996, there were 11 million children in America's 250,000 child-care centers.

■ **Antibiotic overuse.** As a result of this increased exposure, there is more frequent use of antibiotics among youngsters in child care. A study of medication use with children under 3 found that those in child-care centers averaged about 20 days of antibiotic use in a 3-month period, compared with an average of 4 days of use for children the same age who were cared for at home.[11]

■ **Repeated antibiotic use.** Frequent use of antibiotics can affect a child's health in several ways. We now know that antibiotics have tremendous benefits, but also certain limitations. Whenever a child takes these medications, some of the beneficial flora in the digestive tract are destroyed. This increases the tendency to develop yeast infections such as candida, which can compromise a child's digestion and natural immune response.[12] Frequent ear infections can cause scarring of the eardrums, potentially leading to problems in hearing and learning. This research highlights the importance of boosting a child's immunity as a strategy against infectious illness.

■ **Antibiotic-resistance.**   Antibiotic-resistant bacteria can result when the use of antibiotics is high, in settings such as hospitals and child-care centers. A study in Houston discovered that 19 percent of the children in diapers had antibiotic-resistant strains of *E. coli.*[13] Another study compared levels of bacteria in three clusters—two groups of children and one of medical students.[14]

- Children in day care found to have antibiotic-resistant *E. coli*—31 percent
- Children tested at a well-baby clinic with these bacteria—6 percent
- Medical students who tested positive—8 percent

Frequent use of antibiotics can affect a child's health in several ways. Parents of young children who want more information on coping with frequent infections will want to review the sections of the book on strengthening immunity and limiting exposure.

Elementary School Children

Food for Thought

What do kids need to know about germs? By the time children reach elementary school, they have less parental and adult supervision and spend more time in communal spaces, such as buses, crowded classrooms, and school cafeterias. How can they minimize their exposure to germs?

Hand Washing

A number of studies have taught students how to wash their hands and then tracked their school attendance. Typically, the students in the study who consistently washed their hands only missed about half the number of school days, compared with those who didn't have this special emphasis on hand washing.[15,16]

Another study, this one British, tracked an epidemic of hepatitis A that infected 126 students. Practical control measures were instituted, which included advice on good hygiene, supervised hand washing, and additional cleaning in the schools. The epidemic was halted, and there was a low incidence of hepatitis in the schools of that community. Researchers concluded that good hygiene, especially hand washing, remains the most important element in the control of hepatitis A.[17]

A recent study evaluated the use of an alcohol-free hand sanitizer in a public school environment. A 10-week study of 420 elementary school–age children tested the use of a sanitizer spray by students when they first entered the classroom, before eating, and after using the rest room, in addition to normal hand washing with soap and water. Compared with the group that used hand washing only, students using the sanitizer had 42 percent fewer days absence related to illness.

Cafeteria Lunches

We know that the incidence of food poisoning is as high among elementary school children as it is among younger children (see Table 8.3). Although older children have stronger immunity against illness, their exposure tends to be greater. At school they carry their lunch or dine in the school cafeteria. They are also more likely to eat fast food than younger children, when they are with their family or friends.

The research reports outbreaks of a number of different types of food poisoning from food in school cafeterias. These exposures included staph bacteria (staphyloccus), Norwalk-like

Table 8.3 Illnesses That Affect Children 5 to 14 Years Old (Year 2000)

From food and water	*Number of cases reported*
Cryptosporidium infections	629
Hemorrhagic *E. coli* infections	1,083
Hepatitis A	3,009
Salmonella infections	4,751
Shigella infections	5,879
Total	15,351
Insect-borne illness	
Lyme disease	3,489
Airborne illness	
Pertussis (whooping cough)	2,358
Resistant strep pneumonia	188
Tuberculosis	421
Total	2,967

Sources: Data from CDC. Summary of Notifiable Diseases—United States, 2000. *Morbidity and Mortality Weekly Report.* 2002, June 14; 49 (53): 1–102.

virus often associated with shellfish, hepatitis A, and *E. coli.* These outbreaks seem to be relatively isolated incidents.

Researchers also found that the food served in school cafeterias tends to be high in fats and sugar. High sugar intake is of concern because it can reduce white blood cell function, and compromise the activity that protects us against viruses. Our children are exposed to a great deal of bacteria and many viruses in the course of a normal day. We want their immune systems to be in top condition.

Playgrounds

A study by the University of Arizona found that playgrounds rank number one for germ contamination. The researchers

Fifth Disease

Fifth disease is a viral infection that has traditionally been observed as an unimportant rash that may develop in childhood. The rash, caused by human parvovirus (B19), is not usually dangerous to children, but they become carriers for this illness. The virus is spread by exposure to airborne droplets from the nose and throat of infected people. When pregnant women become infected, they are at greater risk for miscarriage or spontaneous abortion. In people with disorders such as sickle-cell disease, which affects red blood cells, fifth disease can result in severe anemia. This virus is also associated with arthritis in adults.

- **Symptoms.** A week or two after exposure, a child may experience a low-grade fever and fatigue. By the third week, a red rash often appears on the cheeks, with the flushed appearance of a slap in the face. The rash may extend to the other parts of the body and tends to fade and reappear. In some cases, the rash may be patchy and appear "lace-like," and it may also itch. Other children may have only vague signs of illness or no symptoms at all.
- **Contagion.** Fifth disease tends to be contagious during the week before the rash appears. By the time the rash is evident, the person is probably no longer contagious. However, someone who is immunosuppressed or who has sickle-cell anemia may be contagious longer.

- **Diagnosis and treatment.** The disease is most often diagnosed on the basis of symptoms. A physician can confirm the diagnosis based on the result of a blood test for antibodies to the parvovirus. (Antibodies are proteins produced by the immune system in response to viruses, bacteria, and other microbes.) The treatment of viral symptoms such as fever, pain, or itching is usually all that is needed. In rare cases, infection by this virus requires hospitalization. People with immune problems may need special medical care, including treatment with immune globulin (antibodies), to help their bodies clear the infection.

SOURCE: CDC. Parvovirus B19 (Fifth Disease). Web site: www.cdc.gov/ncidod/dvrd/revb/respiratory/parvo_b19.htm.

swabbed 800 surfaces in public settings, from pay phones to public restrooms. Playgrounds had the highest potential for germ transmission of all these environments, with evidence of body fluids on 44 percent of the surfaces tested. The researchers' advice? Thorough hand washing!

Whenever people and animals share the same environment, a certain amount of contamination is inevitable. Studies from the United States (Illinois) and cities all over the world had a common finding—the presence of toxacara (worm) eggs in public parks. Toxacara are a type of worm (helminths) that is commonly parasitic to cats and dogs, and conveyed in the stool. In humans, they can cause symptoms ranging from coughing and fever to seizures or more serious conditions. Although the level of contamination varied from study to study, researchers reported on problems in Argentina, Italy, Ireland, Poland, Japan, Germany, and Belgium. Levels of contamination detected ranged from about 3 percent in Argentina to about 64 percent in Italy and Germany.

- In Argentina, the incidence was low in park playgrounds and sandboxes, but higher in housing developments.[18]
- The Italian study also tested those who used the playgrounds and found that positive tests correlated with symptoms of infection.[19]
- The Polish study found that almost half of grassy lawns and sand playgrounds were considered unsanitary.[20]
- In Japan, sandboxes in public parks and playgrounds were more contaminated than those in kindergartens, schools, and children's centers.[21]
- One of the German studies pointed out that the percentage of contaminated samples correlated with the number of dogs in the area.[22]

Swimmers and Water Sports

Swimming Pools

On a hot day, most children will agree that there is nothing quite like a swim. However, the potential for waterborne illness continues to be an issue. Sick children who swim in pools can spread their germs in the water. Healthy children who are swimming in the pool and accidently swallow some of the water are then at risk for illness. Check with the manager of your public pool regarding the level of chlorine used to disinfect the water.

Swimming in Lakes, Streams, and Other Natural Settings

There are a variety of microbes that can infest natural water resources—parasites (such as giardia and cryptosporidium), fecal bacteria (such as *E. coli*), toxic algae, and waterborne viruses. Be sure that the lake or pond has been approved as safe—contact local health authorities and verify the condition of the water.

The Centers for Disease Control tracks outbreaks of illness due to recreational water exposure and contaminated drinking water. A review of outbreaks over a 2-year period, in 1995 and 1996, reported exposure estimated to affect more than 9000 people.[23] Of these, about 8500 cases were involved in two large outbreaks caused by cryptosporidium (a microscopic parasite). Approximately 60 percent of the outbreaks resulted in digestive symptoms such as diarrhea, due to either cryptosporidium or *E. coli*. All cases of *E. coli* were associated with unchlorinated water (in lakes) or low chlorination levels in pools. Pools apparently often contain tiny particles of stool in the water. You can help minimize these problems by not diapering your child by the side of the pool.

Almost 25 percent of the outbreaks resulted in various skin conditions—dermatitis. Of these, seven were associated with the use of hot tubs and two with schistosoma infections contracted in a lake. Six were single cases of meningitis or encephalitis-like illnesses. The report indicated the need for better monitoring of water quality. As a parent, if your child swims, you may want to check with the manager of the pool to determine chlorine levels. You can also check to be sure a pool has been properly sanitized using a simple test that takes about 10 seconds to perform, using test strips (such as those made by GLB or Leisure Time). The strips are inexpensive and can be found at any pool or spa store.

High School and College Age

Fact

Students are more likely to become ill their first year of college than at any other time in their schooling.

Supporting the Immune System

A Doctor's Short Story

Nick and Sandy had been my patients for years. Now they were sitting across from me with their 19-year-old daughter, Lauren.

Table 8.4   Infectious Diseases That Affect Young People 15 to 24 Years Old (Year 2000)

From food and water	*Number of cases reported*
Hemorrhagic *E. coli* infections	631
Hepatitis A	2,098
Salmonella infections	3,366
Shigella infections	1,647
Total	7,742
Insect-borne illness	
Lyme disease	1,632
Airborne illness	
Meningococcal disease	482
Pertussis (whooping cough)	1,247
Tuberculosis	1,623
Total	2,967
Sexually transmitted diseases	
AIDS	1,567
Chlamydia	508,736
Gonorrhea	212,679
Hepatitis B	1,242
Syphilis	1,338
Total	725,562

SOURCE: Data from CDC. Summary of Notifiable Diseases—United States, 2000. *Morbidity and Mortality Weekly Report*. 2002, June 14; 49 (53): 1–102.

Only a few months earlier, Lauren had entered Brown University. Now it was February, and she was on the verge of dropping out. She confided in me, "Dr. Bock, I'm exhausted all the time. I get head aches, and I feel like I have a permanent cold. The worst part is that I can't think straight anymore. I try to study, but I can't remember anything. I can't keep up."

Nicky and Sandy were eager to assure me that Lauren had always been vivacious and industrious. She'd had many interests and friends in high school, a part-time job, and volunteer work. What had gone wrong?

What I see most often in patients is that problems like this tend to develop over time. In September, Lauren was fine—full of energy and enthusiasm. Now she felt depleted and rundown. Getting sick almost always involves a gradual descent, one we're not even aware of until we feel sick. The first changes actually occur in our cells—at the cellular level. When those changes advance to the tissues and organs, we experience them as symptoms. Once we begin to feel ill, we realize that we have a problem.

One of the first systems to become vulnerable is the immune system. Day in and day out, our immunity protects us from germs, toxins, and countless other threats to our health. Immune cells constantly seek out and destroy invading germs in daily skirmishes we can neither see nor feel. However, an overwhelmed immune system is less able to mobilize defenses against these daily assaults. It begins to lose certain battles, and as a result, we get sick.

Think of your immune system as a kettle. The kettle can only hold so much. We're constantly under stress due to viruses, bacteria, pollution, radiation, and other challenges. Yet the immune system can usually handle all this and more. In the context of Lauren's story, it's useful to remember that students in high school and those living away from home for the first time in college often face additional stresses. These include the effects of poor diet, fluctuating hormone levels, psychosocial factors, sleep deprivation, exertion, and smoking. These burdens can add up until one last stress puts us over the top of our "immune system" kettle. Although the result is an illness that can be given a formal diagnosis, there are usually health issues at play much earlier in the disease process.

I see patients every day whose immune systems have been ravaged by a modern lifestyle. I suspected this was what was happening in Lauren's case. Although it would be tempting to describe her situation as a "stress-related disorder," her problems were clearly not caused by psychological stress alone. They were due to the multitude of challenges confronting her immune system. The cumulative effect of her new lifestyle at college had exceeded her immune system's coping capacity. For any of us, lowering some of the challenges can help us tolerate stress without going over our threshold. Lower stress levels make it less likely that our immune system will be overwhelmed or that we'll develop symptoms as a result.

Our conversation made it clear that there were a number of new physical stressors in Lauren's life. She revealed that it was almost impossible to sleep in her dorm. Sometimes she would take a nap during dinnertime when the dorm was quiet, but that was a trade-off since it meant missing dinner. Then she would just grab a snack later on. Her dorm room was below ground and often seemed moldy. Although she wasn't a big partier, she and her friends tended to stay out late socializing. If that wasn't enough stress, all the courses she had were challenging, and she found some of her fellow students academically intimidating.

So Lauren ate poorly, slept poorly, and was under constant pressure. Her "permanent cold" turned out to be an allergic reaction to the mold in her dorm room. Her fuzzy thinking was also due to this allergy. In my experience, mold is one of the allergens that has been associated with problems of alertness and concentration, as well as dizziness, headaches, and sinus pressure. When the results of her tests came back, they confirmed the mold allergy. I knew we couldn't make this allergy disappear, but I was certain that modifying her environment and lowering her total immune burden would bring her some relief. I prescribed nutritional supplements, discussed basic stress management techniques with her, and wrote a letter of medical necessity, recommending that she switch dorm rooms.

Lauren was conscientious about taking her supplements each day and eating better. She still couldn't get much sleep, but she did cut back on the late-night socializing. In about 2 weeks, her head (and her skin) cleared. Once she started to feel better, she felt more like exercising, which helped to lower her stress level. Lauren was able to reverse her downhill slide toward poor health, stayed in college, and ultimately did quite well.

Meningitis

Meningitis is an illness that sometimes causes outbreaks among high school or college students. The research suggests that it is often associated with factors that tend to suppress immunity. Fortunately, only about 500 cases are reported each year, but when it occurs, it can have devastating effects. Meningitis is frequently clustered in small epidemics in college dorms, rather than in isolated cases. For this reason, college students are often vaccinated to protect them against this illness, caused by meningococcal bacteria. About 2200 cases are reported each year in the entire U.S. population, among all ages.

Meningococcal disease typically begins abruptly with a headache, fever, and possible vomiting, as well as rigidity or pain when nodding the head forward. Prompt treatment with antibiotic therapy is effective in more than 90 percent of cases, but if the disease is not treated, it is usually fatal. The incidence of other injuries due to the disease is low—usually hearing deficits or arthritis. However, a life-threatening blood infection can also occur due to these bacteria. In addition, there are occasional cases in which the young person survives but is severely disabled for life.

Although a vaccine is available against meningococcal disease, there are pros and cons to the use of this particular vaccine. Parents will want to confer with their physicians and also with the family member who would be taking the vaccine. The vaccine contains thimerosal, a mercury-based substance that has been linked to neurological damage, which has raised concern among many physicians and parents. A French study (published in 2001) points out that vaccines for this disease are not available for some strains of the bacteria—specifically for meningococcal bacteria type B.[24] The existing vaccine is also reported to be of limited efficacy in infants. Given the potentially serious consequences of the disease, it is vital that families make an informed decision.

Lifestyle Factors and Meningitis

It is important to know that meningococcal bacteria are often found in the nose and throat and are usually "commensal" bacteria—bacteria that live harmlessly in the body without causing infection.[25] Similarly, another form of meningitis is caused by strep bacteria (streptococcus), which are also normally found in the nose and throat in 30 to 60 percent of the population.[26] Following an outbreak of strep-related meningitis in the San Francisco Bay Area, a public health officer pointed out that it is only when the immune system is overtaxed and resistance is low that these bacteria become a problem.

Some recent studies have looked at lifestyle factors that were prevalent in those who contracted meningococcal disease.

Studies conducted independently in England, the Czech Republic, Australia, and France identified a number of factors associated with the disease.

- A British study of meningococcal disease among university students found that they had more than twice the incidence of this disease compared with nonstudents of similar age.[27] An analysis showed that the primary risk factor was eating at the dining hall on campus. Incidence of the disease was much lower at universities that did not provide dining facilities.
- A second British study of university students tracked the percentage of carriers of this bacteria among the student population.[28] Many of the students were carriers—they tested positive for the bacteria but did not have the disease. Over the first week of the semester, the percentage of students who had been exposed went from about 7 percent of the student population to about 23 percent by the fourth day of classes. By December, 34 percent of students tested positive—not for the disease, but as carriers.
- Both Australian[29] and Czech research[30] reviewed cases of meningococcal disease and identified other risk factors:
  - **Conditions that affect the respiratory tract.** Passive or active smoking, exposure to construction dust, environmental contamination, history of snoring or speech problems
  - **Conditions that lower immune function.** Recent illness, or any form of physical or psychological stress, that weakens overall resistance—excessive exposure to cold, alcohol consumption, mental stress, injury, or exertion

- **Conditions that cause increased exposure.** Visits to nightclubs, intimate kissing, sharing a bedroom, overcrowding
- **Beneficial factors.** Active participation in sports, outdoor activity

Protecting Our Children

We can teach our children how to take care of their own health by engaging their interest and empowering them with good information.

1. **Discuss these issues with your health-care practitioner.**
2. **Minimize your child's exposure to germs.**
   - Inform your child about the various infections that kids commonly get.
   - Teach them to decrease their exposure. Good habits are important. We've mentioned some of the studies on the effectiveness of hand washing, which found that washing up before every meal dropped the incidence of illness by 50 percent!

3. **Strengthen your child's immunity.**
   - Let them know the types of behavior that would decrease their resistance, increasing their chance of becoming sick.
   - Provide them with information on building strong immunity. College-age students, for example, can support their health by taking certain key supplements.

These simple steps give power back to both the parent and child (or young adult). It's helpful to know that there is something we can do, rather than just worry.

9

Public Places

IMAGINE THE invisible world that coexists with ours—a world as diverse and complex as the most colorful science fiction—the world of microbes.

We've mentioned that the primary ways germs are conveyed are:

- By airborne transmission
- On surfaces
- Consumed in food and water
- Person-to-person contact

Germs at Work

Let's start where you spend most of your waking hours—at work. Those of you who work in an office may be wondering where most of the germs in your office are lurking. Researchers from the University of Arizona wondered the same thing. They tested about 7000 samples from offices and work cubicles in four major cities.[1] Here's what they learned about where the germs congregate (see Figure 9.1):

Table 9.1   Germs in the Workplace

---

1. Telephone (the worst offender)
2. Desk
3. The handle on the water fountain
4. The handle on the microwave
5. Computer keyboard
6. Elevator button
7. Photocopier start button
8. Photocopier surface
9. Toilet seat
10. Fax machine
11. Refrigerator handle

Researchers point out the gaps in our thinking about what constitutes cleanliness. For example, we don't think twice about eating at our desks, even though the average desk has 100 times more bacteria than a kitchen table and 400 times more bacteria than the average toilet. A small area of the desk or phone can support millions of bacteria—including aggressive species such as *E. coli*, klebsiella, salmonella, staph, and strep. In fact, the area of your desk where you rest your hand holds about 10 million bacteria.[2]

We know one of the major routes of transmission for germs is by contact—by touch. When phones and equipment in an office are shared, if one person has a cold and uses the phone, how likely is it that he or she can pass these germs on? Very likely. The researchers at the University of Arizona also ran a series of tests to track just how germs are transmitted.[3] By the end of the study, they had found that germs in the office could be quickly transferred to hands and face, desktop, drinking cup, computer keyboard, mouse and monitor, doorknob, pen, glasses, and water fountain!

- **How many germs are we typically exposed to?** In another study, the researchers measured the bacteria levels on office coffee mugs.[4] The mugs had bacteria counts ranging from 60 to 400,000 bacteria. When the mugs were cleaned using the grungy sponges on the back of the sink at the office, the bacteria levels climbed higher, producing new counts that ranged from 700,000 to more than a million. The mugs contained scary germs such as hemorrhagic *E. coli* (0157:H7). In addition, 40 percent of the sponges and towels contained coliform bacteria, which are normally found in the digestive tract, but can cause diarrhea.

- **To what degree do we pick up germs on our hands?** Another study at the University of Arizona focused on the role of inanimate objects in the transfer of infectious organisms from one person to another.[5] Common household tasks were carried out with materials covered with microbes. There was little germ transfer from porous materials such as fabric. However, hard surfaces tended to attract the buildup of bacteria, perhaps because a hard surface is a place to which bacteria can cling. Like the findings in the workplace study, the research here showed that the greatest transfer of bacteria occurred by touching the phone. According to the lab tests:

     The phone receiver—38 to 66 percent of the germs on the phone receiver were transmitted to the hand.

     The faucet—28 to 40 percent of the germs on the faucet were transmitted to the hand.

- **Can germs be transmitted to our body if we touch our eyes, nose, or mouth?** When the volunteers' fingertips were coated with the microbes and held up to the mouth, more than one-third of the germs were conveyed to their lips.[6] The percentage of germs that were actually transferred by the fingertips averaged 34 to 41 percent. It is well established that one of the primary routes of infection occurs when we touch our eyes, nose, or mouth with germ-laden hands. The numbers of bacteria transferred to the hands were also significant—up to 106 microbes. Note that with certain types of aggressive bacteria, just 10 microbes are enough to cause infection.

- **The transfer of germs can happen by coming into contact with common objects.** For example, germs can be transferred by headsets. Cold and flu germs can linger on headsets and other objects—thorough cleaning will minimize shared illness. Periodically clean the objects that you handle most frequently.

- **Airborne germs are an issue during cold and flu season.** Opening a window can help clear the air in an office, according to the EPA. Unfortunately, many buildings are designed without easily accessible ventilation, since the windows can't be opened.

- **Do we also take these germs home with us—particularly those we pick up at work or in public spaces?** In another series of tests, the University of Arizona researchers tracked the extent to which germs picked up at work could later be transmitted to the home.[7] Researchers coated office doorknobs with a "tracer" material that mimics the transfer behavior of bacteria. Subjects unknowingly picked up the tracer on their hands as they left the office. Researchers followed the subjects home to study how and where contaminants spread. Typically, on arriving home, most subjects touched about 300 surfaces within 30 minutes. In one example, the subject unknowingly transferred the tracer product to the car door and steering wheel, keys, front doorknob, light switch, TV remote, kitchen counter, kitchen drawer, sink faucet and faucet handles, wallet, and day planner.

Germs in Public Places

Why do we sometimes feel so paranoid about germs in crowded environments and public places? Are our concerns justified? Researchers from Cornell University and their colleagues tested public environments in New York, San Francisco, and Wichita, Kansas.[8] They evaluated the germs on 46 different surfaces, from pay phones to door handles.

Sources of contamination included:

- *E. coli bacteria*, strain 0157:H7, was found on an ATM in the middle of Manhattan. This toxic bacterium has caused several outbreaks of food poisoning and even fatalities. It's most often transmitted in cow manure, so it's not surprising to find it in a meatpacking plant. But on an ATM?
- *Staph aureus*, most well known for its ability to cause wound and respiratory infections in hospitals, was identified on a number of different pay phones in San Francisco. It was also identified at an ATM machine in Nebraska.

Worst Case Scenario

The University of Arizona team evaluated more than 800 public surfaces for levels of general hygiene and the presence of body fluids.[9] The evaluation was performed in three major cities—Tucson, Chicago, and San Francisco. They tested surfaces in a number of public venues. Here's how the various public places scored for hygiene:

- Shopping venues such as retail and grocery stores—44 percent of surfaces failed the hygiene test.
- Public facilities such as playgrounds, health clubs, and restaurants—51 percent failed the test.
- Office environments—46 percent reflected poor hygiene.

Here are the areas they found that were most contaminated by bodily fluids (mucus, urine, stool, blood, etc.) with the percent of contamination:

- Playground surfaces—44 percent
- Bus armrest, handrails—35 percent
- Gym surfaces—28 percent
- Public rest rooms—25 percent
- Shopping cart handles—21 percent
- Chair and seat armrests—21 percent
- Escalator handrails—19 percent
- Customer-shared ballpoint pens—16 percent
- Vending machine knobs—14 percent
- Public telephones—13 percent
- Elevator buttons—10 percent
- Supermarket freezer handles—6 percent

Recreation

Knowing that one in four surfaces failed the general hygiene test, what can you do to protect yourself in public places, like the gym? Just as the doorknob to the office can be covered with germs, so can the grips on the stair climber.[10] The risk of infection at a gym, for example, occurs when someone with a cold or flu wipes his mouth or eyes with his hands and then continues to use the equipment. The virus could be conveyed in the mucus residue. The next person could pick up an infection if she gets some of the mucus on her hands and then touches her eyes. To protect yourself, wash your hands before and after you exercise, and wipe down the machines with disinfectant spray provided by the gym.

Protective Strategies

- Wash your hands often.
- When you can't wash your hands, use waterless antibacterial gel periodically.
- Wipe down your desk, keyboard, and the phone once a day with alcohol and a tissue—or bring alcohol or bleach-based wipes. Just don't let the area get too wet.
- In the kitchen at work, don't let the sponge or cloth sit at the bottom of the wet sink. Put it someplace where it can dry between uses.
- Clean the sponge by running it through a dishwasher or washing machine, or cooking it in the microwave for a minute or two, making sure the sponge is initially damp.
- Better yet, use disposable paper towels.
- To properly sanitize a coffee mug, wash it thoroughly and then rinse it for 30 seconds in water of 170°F or more. Studies have found that one mug in three has bacteria counts over 100, so paper cups could be a good thing.
- Wash your hands as soon as you get home to prevent spreading contaminants to more surfaces and other family members.

Hospitals and Germs

Stepping Up Hospital Safety

Fact

- **The bad news:** Infections acquired in the hospital now affect approximately 2 million people each year, according to the CDC.
- **The good news:** Over the past 10 years, infection rates have actually been decreasing in hospital intensive care units—some nationwide infection rates have dropped by as much as 43 percent.
- **Infection rates** have dropped substantially for all categories of infection.

This chapter takes a brief look at some of the accomplishments of hospitals in controlling infection and risks associated with contagious illness in these environments. We would like to emphasize the exceptional achievements of American hospitals and the Centers for Disease Control and Prevention. We also want to consider concerns people might have when they require surgery or other hospital services.

Accomplishments

First, let's consider how surprisingly safe medical services are. For example:

- **The U.S. blood supply is one of the safest in the world.** In 1985, screening was instituted to identify blood supplies that might contain the AIDS virus. Since that time, only 1 unit of AIDS-contaminated blood slips through the system for about every 500,000 units of blood supplied.[1] Other types of microbes are rarely conveyed by transfusion (i.e., bacteria, spirochetes, or rickettsia), nor does parasitic disease contaminate the blood supply.
- **HIV is rarely transmitted from health care workers to patients in hospitals.** According to the CDC, "Since the onset of the AIDS epidemic almost 20 years ago, only two reports of HIV transmission from an infected health care worker to one or more patients have been published: one in the United States in 1990 and the other in France in 1997."[2] "Epidemiological evidence . . . demonstrates that the risk of (hospital acquired) HIV transmission to patients from an infected provider is extremely low."[3]
- **HIV is rarely transmitted in hospitals from patient to patient.** For example, no cases of patient-to-patient transmission of HIV have been reported from hemodialysis centers in the United States.[4]

Preventing Transmission

In a hospital, germs are transmitted in the same familiar ways they are transmitted in public places or in your home—

airborne transmission, through surface contact, and in body fluids. The medical community has gone to unprecedented lengths to define how these transmissions occur and to avoid their occurrence.

■ **Preventing airborne transmission of fine droplets.** Conditions caused by aggressive airborne bacteria or viruses, particularly tuberculosis, measles, and chicken pox, can be transmitted through fine droplets or dust particles (called droplet nuclei) containing infectious agents. The particles can remain suspended in the air and travel long distances. If the particles are inhaled by a susceptible person, that person could potentially develop an infection. To prevent the spread of these diseases, precautions are taken to prevent airborne transmission by placing an infected patient in a private room, with a closed door and active ventilation to avoid transmission to other patients. In the case of patients with suspected or confirmed tuberculosis, personnel must wear a respirator with a filter one micron or finer that filters out minute particles with an efficiency of at least 95 percent.

■ **Preventing airborne transmission of large droplets.** Large-particle droplets can be transmitted when an infected patient talks, coughs, or sneezes. They can also be transmitted during medical procedures that involve the lungs and airways. Others can become infected if the contaminated droplets land on the mucosal surfaces of the nose, mouth, or eye. Unlike fine airborne particles, the droplets do not remain suspended in the air and do not travel long distances (generally no more than 3 feet). Communicable illnesses that require droplet precautions include bacteria that cause meningococcal infections, such as meningitis, and those that cause severe respiratory illness, such as pneumococcal disease, mycoplasma pneumonia, pertussis, and influenza, as well as mumps, rubella, and fifth disease (parvovirus B19).

- **Avoiding transmission due to physical contact.** Such precautions are intended to prevent the transmission of microbes from an infected patient through direct contact (touching the patient) or indirect contact (touching contaminated objects or surfaces). These precautions also extend to contact with bodily fluids and any germs that could be conveyed through oral-fecal transmission. The patient is typically placed in a private room, health-care workers wear gloves and gowns to minimize trans-mission, and noncritical equipment such as stethoscopes are kept with the patient rather than being used for a number of patients.

- **Protecting the blood supply.** Blood products are another possible means of contagion. The exceptionally low rates of infection reflect the tremendous efforts made by the medical community to maintain a clean blood supply nationwide.

- **Keeping the immune system strong.** Surgical and medical procedures can convey microbes on instruments or equipment. The naturally occurring bacteria within the system may also be transmitted to another area of the body with the potential for infection (this is another good reason to keep your body detoxified). All these situations point out the enormous importance of maintaining a strong immune system.

Risks

In the United States, 3 percent of patients discharged after at least 48 hours in the hospital have some type of infection. In developing nations such as India, that number can be as high as 30 percent. Hospital-acquired pneumonias account for the majority of deaths due to diseases in the hospital. In 2001, in the United States, approximately 103,000 fatalities occurred due to hospital-acquired infections.[5] The health-care costs associated with these infections are nearly $5 billion. It should be pointed out that many of the infections involve patients who have long-term chronic illnesses and weakened immune systems due to illness or injury. Many who contract these infections are taking immunosuppressive drugs as part of treatment, for example in conjunction with transplant surgery.

Types of Infection

The most frequent hospital-acquired illnesses include urinary tract infections, representing about 40 percent of these infections. The large majority of these infections are associated with the use of catheterization. In long-term care facilities, 34 percent of hospital-acquired (nosocomial) infections occur most often in patients with chronic or neurological health issues, who may require catheterization for many months. Pneumonia is the second most frequent infection acquired in a hospital (15 to 20 percent of infections, 250,000 to 300,000 cases per year, at an annual estimated cost of $1.2 to $2.0 billion).[6] These illnesses account for the majority of deaths from hospital infections. Microbes implicated in these infections include *Staph, pseudomonas, klebsiella,* and species of enterobacter.

Approximately 34 million surgical procedures are performed in the United States annually, and between 300,000 and 800,000 infections occur each year as complications of these procedures.[7] The use of hospital equipment also carries the risk of infection, for example in conjunction with procedures such as entubation (the use of specialized tubing to clear the lungs in cases of pneumonia). In addition, medical devices and supplies, such as sutures used to stitch wounds and incisions, have also been found to cause infection.

It has been pointed out that whether a wound infection occurs after surgery depends on a complex interaction among (1) patient-related factors such as host immunity, nutritional status, and the presence or absence of diabetes; (2) procedure-related factors; (3) microbial factors; and (4) antimicrobial (therapy).[8]

Protective doses of antibiotics are used during and after surgery to help destroy bacteria that could cause an infection. Ultimately, the patient's immune system must also play a role. The stronger an individual's immune system, the more successfully he or she can fight the infection. The antibiotic primarily supports this process by destroying many of the harmful bacteria. Those undergoing surgery will want to consider strengthening their body's own defenses.

What You Can Do

Consider adopting personal strategies, outlined in Table 10.1, that reflect to some degree the approaches hospitals use to minimize exposure. There are additional steps you can take to prepare for a hospital procedure and safeguard your health:

- Choose the best possible physician available to you to provide your care. Word-of-mouth is often the best form of recommendation.
- Establish good communication and cooperation with your doctor. Ask about any concerns you might have at a visit scheduled well before the procedure.
- If you have the option of choosing your hospital, participate in that decision. Do your homework. Many

---

Table 10.1   Recommendations for Infection Control

Being Individually Proactive*	Hospital Best Practice+
Be informed	Emphasis on staff education
Monitor the status of your health	Infection surveillance
Practice good hygiene	Interruption of transmission of microorganisms
Minimize your exposure	Prevention of person-to-person spread
Reduce your risk	Modification of risk factors

* Nancy Faass, MSW, MPH.

+ Content from Hospital Infection Control Practices Advisory Committee, Centers for Disease Control and Prevention, Atlanta, GA, 1994.

concerned organizations rate hospitals. This information ranges from statistics kept by health-care organizations to independent ratings in consumer magazines.

- Take a tour of the hospital if it is available. For example, maternity departments often sponsor these tours.
- Be very organized about your hospital stay. Arrive early. Have your support system lined up.
- Learn some good relaxation techniques. You may want to bring a very inexpensive tape recorder with headphones and some tapes you find soothing.
- Strengthen your immune system.

In preparation for the hospital, a program of specific nutrients can speed recovery and reduce discomfort by supporting immune function. Beginning a week or two before surgery, it is helpful to enhance nutrition and supplements.

- **A good high-potency multivitamin.** Most ideal is a formula that includes A and C, B complex, as well as folic acid, calcium, and magnesium, all important for healing. Therapeutic dosages include Vitamin C—1000 to 3000 units per day; vitamin E—400 to 800 units; and zinc—30 to 50 mg a day.

- **Arginine.** This amino acid can be taken in doses of 1000 to 1500 a day. Following surgery, dosages can be increased—1500 to 3000 mg for two weeks to provide additional immune support.
- **Transfer Factor.** These natural immune enhancers aid the body in fighting any possible infection that may occur in conjunction with surgery. Take a standard maintenance dose—three to four capsules a day.

■ **Nutrients to stop.** If you are having surgery, nutrients or herbs that tend to slow blood clotting should be stopped a few days before the procedure and can be reinitiated a few days after surgery. These products include individual doses of vitamin E and herbs such as gingko biloba.

■ **Tune up your diet.** Beginning a few weeks before surgery, you'll want to eat less sugar and have more whole foods, and more organic foods if possible. This style of eating tends to strengthen the immune system and lightens the load of refined foods, additives, and pesticides.

■ **If your digestion is impaired.** You may want to take a multiple amino acid supplement, important for healing, such as Free Aminos or a quality rice protein powder from the health food store.

■ **Additional nutrients following surgery.** You may find these supplements helpful.

- **Proteolytic enzymes.** These contain protease and other protein-digesting enzymes and have been found to significantly improve healing after surgery. Extensive European research has shown that use of a protease supplement can reduce soft-tissue swelling and bruising. Check the particular formula you are using for the dosage.

- **Homeopathics.** Arnica is an exceptional homeopathic remedy for any type of surgical intervention or deep tissue injury. This remedy is available at most health food stores. It is given postoperatively at strengths of 30x, 30c or 200x—see the instructions on the package for dosage.

A Success Story: A Drop in Infection Rates

The setting for this success story is a hospital that is affiliated with a large medical school. The hospital is a tertiary-care facility in a major medical center with 900 beds. In the 32-bed surgical intensive care unit (ICU), an increased incidence of bloodstream infections was identified, exceeding the average infection rate of other hospitals.

In response, three working groups were formed by the hospital to develop new practice guidelines. Products and practices in the ICU were reviewed, and a literature search was performed to review best medical practices. A number of recommendations were adopted by the Infection Prevention and Control Committee involving supplies, practice, and procedures. The working groups also recommended hiring a catheter-care nurse for the surgical intensive care unit. The nurse's responsibilities would include educating the house staff and nursing staff on the clinical practice guidelines, observing actual practices in

A Success Story

providing care, collecting and analyzing outcome data related to bloodstream infections, and providing status reports to the nursing and medical staff.

A *cost-benefit analysis* was presented to the hospital administration to justify hiring the nurse, at a projected salary of $50,000. It was believed a savings of $72,000 could be achieved, which would balance the additional expenditure. The hospital's cost-benefit analysis was effective in securing approval for the position. A registered nurse with 15 years of surgical ICU experience at the hospital was hired. Nine months after joining the infection control team, the nurse reported that 18 fewer bloodstream infections had occurred than in the preceding period the year before, although the hospital's ICU was just as busy. The estimated savings over 9 months was $108,000—and improved quality of life for patients.

When hospital-acquired infections are avoided, everyone wins. Consider the quality of life preserved by minimizing the debilitating effects of infection for the patient. Bloodstream infections—sepsis—can be life-threatening and can also compromise the vital organs. Even after sepsis has been resolved, there can be damage to the kidneys or liver or impaired function. Fewer incidents of resistant infection also means that antibiotics can be used sparingly, hospitalizations are reduced, and there is cost savings to the health care system.

SOURCE: Fran Slater. Cost-effective infection control success story: A case presentation. *Emerging Infectious Diseases*. 2001, Mar.–Apr.; 7 (2). Web site: www.cdc.gov/ncidod/eid/vol7no2/slater.htm.

The Family Pet

The Pet Connection

Fact

- More than 140 million cats and dogs are kept as pets in the United States.[1]
- These pets, as well as other more exotic animals, are found in about 70 percent of U.S. households.
- Pets are associated directly or indirectly with the transmission of at least 30 infectious agents to humans. (See Table 11.1)

Table 11.1 Contagious Illnesses—Pets

	Birds	Cats	Dogs	Reptiles	Best Prevention
Campylobacter	x	x	x		Avoid drinking contaminated water; and exposure to stool of cats, dogs, fowl, or farm animals

Table 11.1 Contagious Illnesses—Pets

	Birds	Cats	Dogs	Reptiles	Best Prevention
Cat scratch disease (*Bartonella henselae*)		x			Keep your cat's nails clipped; immediately wash scratches with soap and water; clean with disinfectant
Cryptosporidium		x	x		Avoid contact with stool; maintain good hygiene and disinfection
H. pylori		x	x		Route of animal transmission unknown
Psittacosis	x				Avoid dust from dried bird droppings of pet birds, parrots, turkeys, and pigeons
Rabies		x	x		Avoid contact with wild animals; keep your pet's rabies vaccine current; if an incident occurs, see your physician immediately (section on rabies has more details)
Ringworm		x	x		Avoid contact with infected animals or objects covered with fungal spores
Roundworm and tapeworm		x	x		Handle animal stool carefully using gloves; wash your hands thoroughly
Salmonella	x	x		x	Take exceptional care in handling reptiles or poultry (see entry on salmonella for specifics)

Table 11.1   Contagious Illnesses—Pets *(continued)*

	Birds	Cats	Dogs	Reptiles	Best Prevention
Toxoplasmosis		X			Use cleanest possible procedure in cleaning the cat litter box

SOURCES OF CONTENT: (1) CDC. Parasitic Pathways—Animals (Zoonotic Diseases). Web site: www.cdc.gov/ncidod/dpd/parasiticpathways/animals.htm. Accessed June 2002. C. Enriquez, N. Nwachuku, and C. P. Gerba. Direct exposure to animal enteric pathogens. *Review of Environmental Health.* 2001, Apr.–Jun.; 16 (2): 117–131. J. S. Tan. Human zoonotic infections transmitted by dogs and cats. *Archives of Internal Medicine.* 1997, Sept. 22; 157 (17): 1933–43.

Overview

Healthy Pets

Infectious conditions carried by pets can be devastating to someone with immune deficiency. The CDC offers advice for patients with HIV who want to continue to keep pets in their home. We felt this advice could also be useful to families who have young children or some other special circumstance.

The basics: Some pets can carry disease-causing germs in their bodies. Others can have fleas or ticks that carry disease-causing germs. Many of the resulting conditions, known as zoonotic (zo-uh-NOT-ick) diseases, could be serious. If you follow recommendations, you can reduce your chance of getting a zoonotic disease. However, anyone who is pregnant or has HIV or AIDS, cancer, an organ transplant, or an immune system disorder will want to pay extra attention to preventive steps. Prevention is also wise when there is a baby, a young child, or an elderly family member in the home, because of the risks associated with certain diseases transmitted by animals.

How Can You Keep Your Pet Healthy?

- Adopt your pet from an animal shelter, or purchase it from a reputable pet store or breeder.
- Have your new pet checked out right away by a veterinarian.
- Keep your pet under a veterinarian's care for regularly scheduled shots and treatment for worms. This reduces the chance that the pet could get sick and pass an infection to you or your family. Since the cost of veterinary care may not be within everyone's reach, the local animal shelter or humane society may have information about low-cost clinics.
- Give your pet a balanced diet. Do not allow it to eat raw food. Don't let it drink out of the toilet.
- Wear rubber gloves when cleaning aquariums, cages, or litter boxes.
- Clean your pet's living area at least once a week. Bury or flush feces, or place them in a plastic bag and put the bag in the trash. Clean litter boxes daily.
- To prevent infectious diseases that may cause birth defects such as toxoplasmosis, pregnant women should not change cat litter boxes.
- A child's sandbox can become a cat's litter box, so cover it when not in use. Areas that have been contaminated with dog or cat feces should be off-limits to children—not only at home but also in public areas such as parks or playgrounds. And because toddlers naturally explore their environment, teach children not to eat dirt, which can expose them to parasites.

- Wash your hands with soap and water and use a nailbrush after handling or cleaning up after animals, including reptiles. Teach your children to do the same.

Campylobacter

Campylobacter is the most common bacterial cause of diarrheal illness in the United States, estimated to affect more than 2 million people each year. Symptoms include diarrhea, cramping, abdominal pain, headache, fatigue, and fever that typically begins 2 to 5 days after exposure. Diarrhea may be bloody and can be accompanied by nausea and vomiting. Some of those infected have no symptoms at all. The illness typically lasts about a week. These are bacteria found in the reproductive organs, intestinal tract, and mouth of both animals and humans.

Diagnosis and Treatment

Diagnosis can be made through a stool culture. It's important to drink plenty of fluids as long as the diarrhea lasts. In more severe cases, antibiotics can be used, and can shorten the duration of symptoms.

In rare cases, long-term consequences can result from a campylobacter infection. Guillain-Barré syndrome is a rare disease that affects the nerves of the body, which occurs as an autoimmune condition when the immune system is "triggered" to attack the nervous system. The condition can lead to paralysis that lasts several weeks and usually requires intensive care. It is estimated that about 1 in every 1000 reported campylobacter infections leads to Guillain-Barré syndrome. As many as

40 percent of the cases in this country may be triggered by campylobacter infection.

The Animal Connection

Pets are a frequent source of this illness, particularly dogs and puppies. Among dogs with diarrhea, 28 percent were found to harbor campylobacter. Other potential sources of human infection due to campylobacter include poultry, cattle, sheep, and pigs.

- *Campylobacter jejuni* grows best at the body temperature of a bird, and it seems to be well adapted to birds, which carry it without becoming ill.
- Some people have acquired their infection from contact with the infected stool of an ill dog or cat. To avoid contamination, always wash your hands with soap after handling animals, and particularly whenever there is contact with pets or pet feces.
- Surface water and mountain streams can become contaminated from infected feces of cows or wild birds.
- Poultry are another major source of contamination, including improper food handling of raw poultry or eating undercooked (or raw) poultry meat. Even one drop of juice from raw chicken meat can transmit infection. Many chicken flocks are silently infected with campylobacter—the chickens are carriers of the organism but show no signs of illness, and the contagious bacteria can be easily spread from bird to bird. When an infected bird is slaughtered, campylobacter can be transferred from the intestines to the meat. More than half of the raw chicken in the U.S. market has campylobacter bacteria.

Prevention

- Thoroughly wash your hands whenever you have contact with an animal and before eating or handling food.
- Practice safe food handling. This is key since poultry is a reservoir for this illness. (See Chapter 4 for more information on food preparation.)
- Be sure to obtain prompt testing and treatment for sick animals, including those that develop diarrhea.

Cat Scratch Disease

The Pet Connection

This disease, caused by the bacteria *Bartonella henselae*, occurs after exposure through a cat bite, a cat scratch, or the infected cat's fleas. Cats serve as a major reservoir for this illness and are contagious through their saliva. The bacteria that cause cat scratch disease can also cause a bacterial infection of the bloodstream— bacteremia. The fleas removed from these cats may also contain the infectious agent, and bites from these fleas can transmit the disease. In the United States, up to 50 percent of cats tested have antibodies against this organism, which indicates they have been exposed to this bacteria and could be carriers.[2]

Symptoms and Treatment

Typically, this is a benign infection in children; the primary symptom is swollen lymph glands. Even when these bacteria can be identified in the lymph node tissue, the lab cultures often come back negative, for reasons that are not yet under-stood. In most cases, the disease is self-limited, and complete resolution occurs within 2 to 6 months. Systemic disease and chronic, relapsing illnesses have been known to occur. AIDS patients may develop skin lesions as a result of this infection. Bartonella infections can also be transmitted by a tick bite. These infections tend to be quite invasive, causing symptoms similar to Lyme disease—fatigue, headaches, arthralgias, and swollen glands. It is encouraging to know that Bartonella infec-tions can be successfully treated with antibiotics such as doxy-cycline, azithromycin, or avelox.

Prevention

- Immediately wash any scratch with soap and water and then disinfect it with alcohol, hydrogen peroxide, or Betadine iodine solution.
- Keep your cat as generally healthy as possible.
- Keep the cat's nails trimmed short to minimize the risk of scratches.

Cryptosporidium

Cryptosporidium is a diarrheal disease caused by a microscopic parasite that can live in the intestine of humans and animals and is passed in the stool of an infected person or animal. The parasite is protected by an outer shell that allows it to survive outside the body for long periods of time. In the environment, this outer shell makes it very resistant to chlorine disinfection. During the past 20 years, cryptosporidium has become recog-nized as one of the most common causes of waterborne disease in humans in the United States—due to contaminated drinking water and also exposure during recreational water sports. The parasite is found in every area of the United States and throughout the rest of the world.

Symptoms and Treatment

Symptoms include diarrhea, loose or watery stool, stomach cramps, upset stomach, and a slight fever. Symptoms generally begin 2 to 10 days after being infected. Some people have no symptoms. In those with average immune systems, symptoms usually last about 2 weeks—the symptoms may go in cycles, with periods of improvement and then relapses. This illness can be devastating to people who are immune-compromised. Cryptosporidium can also be very contagious.

The Animal Connection

Cryptosporidium lives in the intestine of humans or animals. It may be found in soil, food, water, and surfaces that have been contaminated with the feces from infected humans or animals. It can be spread in lakes, rivers, springs, ponds, or streams that are contaminated with sewage or feces from humans or animals. For example, in the San Francisco Bay Area, a local reservoir for drinking water was found to harbor cryptosporidium from cattle manure. The cattle were grazing on the grassy hills near the reservoir, and the rainwater runoff from the hillside contaminated the reservoir. In addition, millions of microbes can be released in a single bowel movement from an infected human or animal, so one person in a swimming pool or lake can potentially infect many others. One can become infected after accidentally swallowing the parasite in drinking water or while swimming.

The infection can also be contracted by ingesting food or drinking water that contains traces of the microbe. Cryptosporidium is not spread by contact with blood.

Although cryptosporidium can infect anyone, this parasitic organism flourishes under conditions of compromised immune function. As a result, those who are vulnerable are more likely to develop serious illness.

Testing and Supportive Care

Diagnosis involves antibody testing or stool antigen testing. This type of evaluation is available through labs that specialize in these tests and can be ordered through an integrative physician. There is currently no effective medication. Most people with a healthy immune system will recover on their own. Young children and pregnant women may be more susceptible to the dehydration resulting from diarrhea and should drink plenty of fluids while ill. Rapid loss of fluids because of diarrhea can be life threatening in babies; parents should consult their health-care provider about fluid replacement therapy options for infants and small children. Antidiarrheal medicine may help slow down diarrhea, but be sure to consult with your health-care provider before taking it.

Prevention

Practice good hygiene:

- Wash your hands thoroughly with soap and water after using the toilet and before handling or eating food. If you have diarrhea, also use a nailbrush and disinfect your hands with alcohol afterward.
- If there is an infant in the house or if you work in day care, wash your hands after every diaper change even if you are wearing gloves.

- Protect others by not swimming if experiencing diarrhea. Don't allow children in diapers to use public pools or lakes whether they have diarrhea or not.

Avoid Water That Might Be Contaminated

- Avoid swallowing water in a pool or other recreational swimming environment.
- Avoid drinking untreated water from shallow wells, lakes, rivers, springs, ponds, streams, or fountains in public parks. Always carry your own water.
- Avoid drinking untreated water during communitywide outbreaks of diseases caused by contaminated drinking water. In the United States, nationally distributed brands of bottled water or carbonated soft drinks are considered safe.

H. Pylori

This spiral bacterium is associated with over 90 percent of cases of duodenal ulcers and 70 to 80 percent of stomach ulcers. These bacteria can interfere with the natural acid production of the stomach in order to establish the infection. This impairs digestion and also leaves the body less protected against infection since stomach acid is one of the body's main defenses against microbes. *H. pylori* infections can cause inflammation and discomfort or pain. In addition, the chronic inflammation that results can set the stage for heart disease or gastric cancer. At least 23 species of *H. pylori* have been identified. Although no clear routes of transmission between animals and humans have been confirmed, there are numerous indicators of this transmission.

Diagnosis and Treatment

Diagnosis is made on the basis of a biopsy, blood test, or a breath test. Successful treatment requires combination drug therapy, including the use of two antibiotics, as well as other medication. Over the past 10 years, *H. pylori* bacteria have become more resistant to an increasing number of medications. This is a worldwide trend. For those who want to try an alternative treatment before going on antibiotics, we have had success with a natural regimen using a product called gum mastic taken three times a day, sometimes in combination with olive leaf extract. Bentonite, taken daily, has also been found beneficial in some cases.

The Animal Connection

H. pylori has been detected in housecats suffering from gastritis comparable to that of humans. Contact with dogs has also been identified as a risk factor. Links to sheep and cattle have also been suggested in the research literature.

> *So far, no non-human or environmental reservoir has been proven, nor has any definitive means of transmission been established.* H. pylori *has been found in monkeys and in laboratory cats, and there have been reports of other gastric* Helicobacter-*like organisms in those species as well as in dogs. More studies will be needed to determine whether* H. pylori *naturally colonizes domestic dogs and cats and whether these pets can transmit* H. pylori *or other animal-associated* Helicobacter *to humans. Recent evidence from Chile supports the theory of human colonization by* Heli-

cobacter *species originally found in animals. In those studies, investigators demonstrated genetic evidence for the presence of several species of animal-associated intestinal* Helicobacter *in the gall bladders of individuals with chronic cholecystitis [inflammation of the gallbladder].*[3]

Prevention

Cats in particular are strongly suspected to be a carrier of *H. pylori.* Individuals who have allergies or low resistance to illness may want to consider not sleeping with their pets. Since the mechanism of transmission has not yet been determined, we can only recommend maintaining good immunity, healthy pets, and good general hygiene.

Chlamydia Psittaci

Several strains of the bacteria *Chlamydia psittaci* can cause respiratory illness—it can cause psittacosis in humans and birds and pneumonitis in cattle, sheep, swine, cats, goats, horses, and other mammals. In birds, psittacosis can cause respiratory problems, eye infection, diarrhea, weight loss, or lethargy, as well as sudden death.

In humans, psittacosis symptoms can include respiratory problems, muscle aches, fever, headache, and fatigue. This condition has an incubation period of about 10 days, with variable symptoms. It usually results in a week of illness.

In humans, the condition is diagnosed with a blood test that evaluates antibody levels (immune "artillery" in the blood that indicate the presence of infection). Diagnosis is much more difficult in birds because they do not produce antibodies and stool tests can be unreliable. Both birds and humans can be treated with antibiotics, in addition to supportive therapy.

It is important to seek treatment immediately and resolve the condition. Psittacosis can cause a serious prolonged illness in anyone who has a vulnerable or immature immune system, such as a young child.

Prevention

The disease can be transmitted through direct contact with birds, breathing in feather dust, breathing dust from fecal buildup in a birdcage, or by direct contact with bird droppings. Avoid dust from the dried bird droppings of parrots, turkeys, and pigeons. Also avoid environments that have extensive residues of bird fecal matter.

If you have pet birds:

- Clean the cage regularly to prevent the buildup of droppings.

- Do not kiss your bird or let it nibble your face.

- Provide a healthy diet and suitable housing for your pet.

- In addition, birdkeepers in dusty aviaries should wear dust masks.

Rabies

Rabies is a disease caused by a virus found in the saliva of infected animals. It can be transmitted to pets and humans through bites or in some cases by the contamination of an open cut with the saliva of an infected animal. Wild animals accounted for 93 percent of all reported cases of rabies in 2000.[4] Treatment is critical for a person who has been infected. *Once the symptoms of the disease appear, the virus can be fatal and there is no known cure.*

Treatment

Effective human rabies vaccines have been developed in case of exposure due to an animal bite. Immunoglobulin transfusions are also available—these contain natural immune factors that can be given to increase immunity following exposure. Each year, an estimated 18,000 people (such as lab workers) receive rabies pre-exposure prophylaxis, and an additional 40,000 receive post-exposure treatment. There have been no vaccine failures in the United States when post-exposure treatment was given promptly and appropriately. *Note that treatment must be given soon after exposure to be effective.*

Preventive Measures

The incidence of rabies cases nationwide is monitored by the CDC. In the year 2000, more than 7000 cases of rabies occurred, up about 4 percent from the year before. Of these, about one-third were due to raccoons and one-third to skunks. There was an increase in cases involving rabid skunks, foxes, and bats, as well as dogs and domestic sheep and goats. An animal infected with rabies may show no visible symptoms for several days. Therefore, as prevention, avoid contact with unfamiliar animals.

- Enjoy wild animals from afar, but do not handle them, feed them, or unintentionally attract them with open garbage cans or litter.
- Never adopt wild animals or bring them into your home.
- Do not try to nurse sick animals to health. Instead, call animal control or an animal rescue agency.
- Teach children never to handle unfamiliar animals, whether wild or domestic, even if they appear friendly.
- Prevent bats from entering living quarters or occupying public spaces since they might come in contact with people and pets and are potential carriers for rabies.
- When traveling abroad, avoid direct contact with wild animals, and be especially careful around dogs in developing countries. Rabies is a common disease in Asia, Africa, and Latin America, where dogs are the major reservoir. Rates of rabies in some developing countries are 100 times higher than those in the United States. Tens of thousands of people die of rabies each year in these countries. Before traveling abroad, consult with a health-care provider about the risk of exposure and protective measures to be taken.

Pet Care

- Keep vaccinations up to date for all dogs, cats, and ferrets.
- Keep your pets under direct supervision so they do not come in contact with wild animals.
- Call your local animal control agency to remove any stray animals from your neighborhood.

- Spay or neuter your pets to help reduce the number of visits from unwanted pets that may be unvaccinated.

Coping with an Animal Bite

Since rabies can be fatal, if an animal bite is suspected, be sure to call the Health Department. Whenever anyone is bitten, it's important to determine if the dog's rabies shots were up to date or if the animal might be rabid. Dog owners are sometimes dishonest about whether their pet's shots are up to date. Don't leave your child's health to chance.

1. Check the dog's collar to see if it's rabies shots are to date.
2. If the animal is captured or killed, call the Health Department. They will pick up the animal and monitor it or autopsy it for rabies.
3. If the animal gets away, call your doctor or the state health department immediately for treatment advice.
4. If you suspect that your own pet is rabid, it can be monitored by the Health Department to determine whether or not it is.
5. Remember, anyone who is bitten has a limited time period in which to get an injection to protect them against rabies.

Ringworm

Ringworm is classified as a dermatophyte (der-MA-to-fite). This surprisingly common fungus causes superficial infections of the skin, hair, or nails. Although there are about 35 species of fungus that affect household pets, *Microsporum canis* is the primary cause of ringworm in cats, dogs, and humans, in about 95 percent of cases. It is also associated with a form of ringworm of the scalp (called *Tinea capitis*) that causes patches of baldness in children who have contracted the fungus from their pet. The fungus is characterized by circular scaly lesions or patches of hair loss. Puppies, kittens, and children are most prone to these infections, which can be transmitted through contact with other animals or their environment.

Diagnosis

Pets carrying this fungal infection may or may not have symptoms of ringworm. Those clearly infected will tend to have a patchy coat. Dogs are more likely to also have inflammation. Diagnosis can be made by the vet through a skin culture. Some cases may resist treatment because the animal can continue to harbor the fungus even though it has no symptoms, so periodic testing may be necessary.

Treatment

The elimination of ringworm involves the use of antifungal creams on animals and humans. In severe cases, an oral antifungal medication is also necessary. For stubborn cases, an integrative approach would also involve an antiyeast program to decrease overall sensitivity to the fungus. Handling the animal may involve applying topical ointments, using an antifungal wash weekly, and continuing treatment for at least 21 days. You'll want to wear gloves during this procedure. Keeping the animal clean and healthy will also help to minimize recurrences. Infected animals should be quarantined from animals that are not infected and from people.

Environmental Measures

It's important to clean and disinfect the living environment to prevent reinfection. A solution of bleach (1 part bleach to 10 parts water) can be effective. Thorough and frequent vacuuming should be performed to clear animal hair and dander from bedding, clothing, and carpets, as well as air-conditioning and heating filters. Wear rubber gloves, and shower and wash clothes after the job is done.

Roundworms and Tapeworms

These worms can be transmitted from both cats and dogs, as well as other animals. Due to limited availability of lab testing that focuses on parasitic infection, these conditions are probably vastly underdiagnosed and underreported. *Taenia* (tapeworm) species related to animals include beef, pork, and fish tapeworm, as well as *Dipylidium caninum*, the common tapeworm of cats and dogs. Ascaris are roundworms that can also infect animals and humans. These and other related infectious agents are classified as helminths (worms). Any of these species can be transmitted to humans.

Symptoms

Ascaris (roundworms) are highly infectious and can cause abdominal pain, nausea, and digestive disturbances. In large numbers, worms can actually cause a blockage. Intestinal worms tend to migrate into the ducts of the liver. Ascaris can trigger allergies that can persist years after the infection has cleared.

Taenia solium (pork tapeworm) seldom causes appreciable symptoms, in contrast to other types of parasites that may cause symptoms. The intestine may be irritated at sites of attachment. In some cases, abdominal discomfort, chronic indigestion, and diarrhea may occur.

Diagnosis and Treatment

See your vet regarding your pet's diagnosis. Note that tapeworm eggs are rarely released into animal feces and are therefore not usually detected by the routine fecal exams that vets perform. Although cats and dogs are not usually ill as a result of a tapeworm infection, you may see signs of the infection, such as grains that resemble rice clinging to the animal's bottom. If your dog is infected, it may experience vomiting.

Human diagnosis is best performed through stool evaluation that includes testing for antigens (chemical evidence of the parasite, which can be detected through lab work). Antibody testing is another relatively effective form of testing. Both these types of evaluation have a better track record than routine-type stool testing.

The vet can prescribe worm medication for your dog or cat. Human treatment is achieved through antiparasitic medication prescribed by a doctor who is experienced in the treatment of parasites. It is important that all people and pets in the household be treated simultaneously to break the cycle of transmission. A repeated round of medication may be needed several weeks later. Scrupulous hygiene must be maintained during this period. There is also value in having periodic checkup evaluations.

Prevention

- Thorough vacuuming and good hygiene are important.
- Don't let pets lick your face, and don't kiss them.
- Never let cats sit on tables or other surfaces where food or dishes are kept.
- You will probably want to avoid having your pets sleep in your bed.
- Since fleas can be a carrier for cat and dog tapeworms, flea control is one of your best strategies.

Salmonella

Salmonella is a common infectious agent that has more than 2000 different species. It has been identified in poultry and eggs (an estimated 2 million eggs a year are believed to be contaminated with salmonella bacteria). Animals such as swine, cattle, and sheep also serve as carriers for the disease; and sometimes, have no symptoms even though they have the disease.

The Pet Connection

Although food-borne salmonella is the major form of transmission in humans, pets are also an important source of exposure. For example, it has been found that between 20 and 27 percent of dogs have been infected, usually with a blood type similar to the type affecting humans. Infections in animals may have few apparent symptoms, but the bacteria can cause fever, diarrhea, or spontaneous abortion.

A review of the medical literature suggests that birds and reptiles are even more likely to serve as reservoirs for this infection.

Birds known to carry the disease include baby chicks, duck-
lings, and pheasants. Salmonella infections have been linked to
reptiles kept as pets, such as snakes, lizards, iguanas, komodo
dragons, and tortoises. These infections have also been identified in wild and zoo animals.

Diagnosis and Treatment

Salmonella is not normally an inhabitant of the human digestive tract, except during infection. It can cause diarrhea, which
may be severe. *Salmonella typhi* (which causes typhoid fever) is
also invasive and can cause systemic infection. With typical salmonella infections, most patients require no therapy. If systemic illness occurs, the most potentially effective antibiotic
therapy can be determined through laboratory testing. In the
United States, treatment with antibiotics is usually successful.

Prevention

- Optimal hygiene habits and safe food handling.
- Frequent hand washing.
- When choosing pets, if there are young children in
  the house or a family member who is pregnant or
  immune-compromised, it may be good to avoid
  amphibious pets such as reptiles or turtles.

Toxoplasmosis

This is one of the most common protozoan infections of
humans and animals, carried by cats and a broad range of inter-
mediate hosts. It has been documented in about 300 species of

mammals and 30 species of birds. Most infections cause no symptoms in those who are healthy, but they can be life threatening in someone who is immunocompromised. Toxoplasmosis can be devastating to a developing fetus.

The Pet Connection

Toxoplasmosis lives within the cell. Its natural host is the cat. The microbe resides within the digestive tract, transmitting infection through the stool. It can also be ingested in raw or undercooked meat. In adult humans, it can cause mild flu-like symptoms and possibly enlarged lymph glands. However, this illness can have serious consequences for a pregnant woman and her unborn child. Once the infection is established, it can cross the placenta and be transmitted to the fetus. As a result, there may be damage to the eyes or the brain or even death.

Cats become infected by ingesting food that contains the toxoplasma cysts or meat containing the cysts. It has been estimated that an area about 3 feet square (a square meter) can harbor about 200 to 800 cysts. The cysts can remain contagious even after more than 300 days in sunlight and 400 days in the shade. Infection in kittens is more common than infection in adult animals and may occur once the kitten begins hunting birds and rodents. As a result, young cats represent a great risk for infection. Pregnant women will want to take this into account in order to minimize their risk.

Treatment and Prevention

These conditions can be treated with medication. They are best avoided by practicing good hygiene and thoroughly cooking meat. If a pregnant woman is in the household, she should not be responsible for cleaning up the cat litter box since microbes can be transmitted on dust and any surfaces that have not been disinfected.

Avoiding Germs from Animals

Which Efforts Count Most?

What Is the Most Serious Disease That Animals Can Transmit to People?

The rabies virus is the most serious acute illness that animals transmit. Cats, as well as dogs, should be immunized against rabies. The number of rabies cases in the United States has been drastically reduced. However, rabies is still found in wild animals and more than 90 percent of rabies cases are now due to bites by wild animals.

What about Having a Wild Animal as a Pet?

In general, wild animals do not make good pets because they are not tame and do not adapt well to living in a house. They also carry a greater potential for rabies. If you elect this type of pet, make sure you know about any special needs the animal has and any diseases it can transmit. Then have it carefully checked out by your vet. Generally speaking, animals that carry a greater risk of disease include strays, animals with diarrhea or other signs of illness, and wild or exotic animals, including monkeys. Due to risk of salmonella, turtles and reptiles, such as snakes and iguanas, are not recommended for young children.

What to Do When an Animal Scratch or Bite Occurs

Each year almost 800,000 persons are bitten by dogs or cats and require medical attention. Never approach an unfamiliar animal. When bitten or scratched, always:

- Wash the area with soap and water, preferably antibacterial soap.
- Apply antibacterial medication such as Betadine soap, hydrogen peroxide, or alcohol.
- Bandage the wound, and consider getting medical attention.
- If there is any suspicion of rabies, see a health-care practitioner immediately, since rabies is potentially fatal.
- Be sure to teach your children to tell you about any animal bite or scratch they receive.

How Can We Minimize Our Exposure?

- Wear gloves when gardening.
- Cover children's sandboxes when not in use.
- If you have a dog, make sure your children wear shoes when in the yard or garden.
- Remove all of your pet's deposits from the garden on a daily basis.
- If your pet is unwell, especially if it has diarrhea or skin disease, consult your vet. If the diarrhea lasts for more than 1 or 2 days, ask the veterinarian to check the pet for infections. If you are immune compromised, have a friend or relative take your pet to the veterinarian.

- If you are immune compromised, pregnant, or have a small child in the household, don't get a pet that is younger than 6 months old. There is a higher potential for communicable illness, such as worms, in young animals.
- If you are getting a pet from a pet store, animal breeder, or animal shelter (pound), check the sanitary conditions and license of the sources. Select a pet that is healthy-looking—and still have it checked out by your veterinarian.
- The same precautions apply for children as for adults. However, children tend to snuggle more with their pets and are more vulnerable to being scratched or bitten. Some pets, like cats, may bite or scratch to get away from children. Teach children how to handle animals and supervise their hand washing to prevent infections.
- If you use an insecticide such as flea powder, be sure to follow instructions carefully. Both adults and children with allergies or asthma should avoid exposure to these insecticides.

What about the Litter Box?

- Animal feces are a primary source of disease transmission.
- Keep the box away from the kitchen and eating areas.
- Change the litter box daily. Pregnant women should get someone else to do this.
- Use disposable plastic liners and change them each time you change the litter.

- Don't dump litter! If inhaled, the resultant dust could infect you. Instead, gently seal the plastic liner with a twist tie and place in a plastic garbage bag for disposal.
- Disinfect the litter box once a month by wiping it out and then filling it with boiling water and letting it stand for five minutes. No other disinfecting method seems to kill the toxoplasmosis organism.
- Wear gloves and a dust mask (you can get these at the hardware store). Always wash your hands after cleaning the litter box.
- Think about having your pet's feces checked by your veterinarian from time to time for parasitic diseases such as toxoplasmosis—especially if your pet goes outside.
- Remember that animal droppings in flower beds or sandboxes present the same health risks as they do in a litter box.

What Should I Feed My Pet?

The following are ways you can prevent your pet from catching diseases that may be passed on to humans:

- Feed your pet only reputable pet foods.
- Never feed your pets raw meat or unpasteurized milk.
- Don't let your pet eat its own or other animals' feces.
- Don't let your pet drink from the toilet bowl or rummage through the garbage.
- Don't let your pet hunt other animals. Cats can catch toxoplasmosis from eating infected birds or rodents. If you have an outdoor cat, think about placing a double bell on its collar to help warn potential prey.

If you have a farm cat who hunts rodents, you should have its feces examined regularly for signs of infection.
- Keep your dog on a leash to prevent scavenging.

What about Other People's Animals?

There have been cases of schoolchildren being infected with Q fever from handling newborn baby goats. Parents and teachers should be careful on field trips to farms to not let children touch or handle newborn animals or the byproducts of the birthing process (blood, afterbirth, body fluids, etc.). Children visiting petting zoos have become infected by *E. coli* bacteria after contact with manure on the animals or in the environment. They should be warned not to put their hands in their mouths, and they should wash their hands right after their visit, and *before* they eat or handle food.

The Benefits of Having a Pet

We believe that in most cases the positive benefits of having a pet far outweigh the negatives. The companionship of an animal can definitely be mood-enhancing. The emotional enrichment that animals provide can counter the isolation and loneliness that many people tend to feel. We know from a great many studies that this emotional nurturing is important to one's health and quality of life. We've focused on the risks here. However, if you just take the most basic precautions described in this chapter, that should afford you a reasonable level of protection. Then you can enjoy the immensely positive experience of the companionship of a pet.

The Safe Traveler

TRAVEL CAN BE one of the most exciting experiences of our lives, and yet occasionally it can pose serious risks to our health. Getting sick when one travels is no fun. Bringing home illness is equally unpleasant—particularly if exotic viruses or bugs linger.

We can minimize our exposure in some situations, so it's useful to know as much as possible about where we're going and what the risks are. (For example, do harmful parasites infest the scenic rivers, making swimming unwise?) In other situations, such as air travel, our control is limited. We breathe the same air as everyone else on the plane. In those cases, building up one's immunity is one of the most effective strategies. Here natural medicine can make a contribution. We'll provide an overview of some of the most important travel issues and then offer steps you can take to make travel healthier.

Immunizations

Specific vaccines are recommended on a country-by-country basis, depending on the most prevalent diseases in a particular area. The most current resources regarding vaccine recommendations are the web site and publications of the Centers for Disease Control and Prevention. On the web, the CDC's site can be accessed at www.cdc.gov. See the Resources section at the back of the book for the CDC's publications and other useful information as well. The primary vaccinations are listed in Table 12.1. Note that the strongest of the vaccines (the "live" vaccines) should be taken 3 weeks apart to minimize reactions. This requires advanced planning and scheduling, so that your body has time to adjust and recoup after each vaccination.[1]

Table 12.1 Specific Immunizations Related to Travel

The strongest vaccines are live vaccines that should be taken at least 3 to 4 weeks apart, including those for:

- Measles, mumps, rubella
- Polio (oral)
- Tuberculosis
- Typhoid
- Yellow fever

Additional vaccines, appropriate to particular environments, include those for:
- Cholera
- Diphtheria (typically a childhood vaccination)
- Hepatitis A
- Hepatitis B
- Influenza
- Japanese encephalitis (related to West Nile virus)
- Meningococcal meningitis
- Plague
- Rabies
- Tetanus

SOURCE: Information from CDC. *Health Information for International Travel, 2001–2002.* McLean, VA: International Medical Publishing, 2001, pp. 19, 20.

Building Immunity

It's important to support your immune system with nutritional supplements when you travel. A few days before you travel, you'll probably want to begin your program of immune support. Continue this during your trip and also take the supplements for a few days after you return home, just to be sure. If you are going to be traveling overseas or if you feel run-down, begin a week before and end a week after your trip. Here are some nutritional supplements we consider essential when we travel:

Supporting Your Immune System When You Travel

Nutritional supplements we consider essential when traveling or flying include:

- **A good high-potency, balanced multiple vitamin.**
- **Vitamin C.** Typically taken 3,000 to 9,000 mg. (Be sure you know your bowel tolerance level before you travel—high doses of vitamin C can cause diarrhea.)
- **Transfer Factor.** Take 6 capsules per day.
- **Immune-enhancing polysaccharides.** For added support, take Immpower, Chinese mushrooms, or Transfer Factor Plus, which includes immune supportive polysaccharides. (See the Resources section for additional information.)

Protection for the Digestive Tract

The digestive tract is vulnerable to germs in food and water. The best strategy is to minimize exposure by eating very prudently while strengthening the defenses of the digestive system with key supplements such as:

- **Colostrum.** This is an extract containing the immune-enhancing properties of "first" milk, extracted from cow's milk. For travel, typically 2 capsules are taken daily.
- **Bismuth (PeptoBismol) or Gastromycin.** Bismuth is a mineral that is usually quite well tolerated and that can help prevent infection. The CDC indicates that "bismuth . . . taken as the active ingredient of PeptoBismol has decreased the incidence of diarrhea by about 60 percent in several . . . studies."[2] However, products containing bismuth should not be taken for more than three weeks consecutively. Note that bismuth is not appropriate for children with chicken pox or flu, very young children, and anyone with an aspirin allergy or taking therapeutic doses of aspirin.
- **Probiotics.** These supplements are best taken after meals or on an empty stomach. Look for a high-potency formula that does not require refrigeration such as Kyo-Dophilus. If you will have access to refrigeration, you can use a formula that contains acidophilus, bifidus, and beneficial yeast such as Co-biotic.

Minimizing Your Risk

Food Safety

You can also conserve immune defenses by reducing your exposure. The CDC points out that not all countries have high standards of food hygiene. The CDC recommends that those who are immune-compromised take special care abroad, particularly in developing countries, by following these basic rules:

- Do not eat uncooked fruits and vegetables unless you can peel them. Avoid salads.
- Eat cooked foods while they are still hot.
- Boil all water before drinking it. Drink only canned or bottled drinks or beverages made with boiled water. Use only ice made from boiled water.

To sum it up, the safest foods include steaming-hot foods, fruits you peel yourself, bottled and canned processed drinks, and hot coffee or tea.

At home and abroad:

- Order all food well done. If meat is served pink or bloody, send it back to the kitchen for more cooking. Fish should be flaky, not rubbery, when you cut it.
- Be sure eggs are always well cooked. Fried eggs should be cooked on both sides, and scrambled eggs should be cooked until they are not runny. Do not order foods that may contain raw or lightly cooked eggs, such as Caesar salad or hollandaise sauce. If you aren't sure about the ingredients in a dish, ask your waiter before you order.

- Do not order any raw or lightly steamed fish or shellfish, such as oysters, clams, mussels, sushi, or sashimi. All fish should be cooked until done.
- Avoid seafood that carries the risk of toxins from fish or shellfish—these toxins are not destroyed by cooking. Currently, barracuda should always be avoided, but a wide range of tropical reef fish and species such as red snapper, grouper, and sea bass also contain toxins at unpredictable times. The risk is present in all subtropical and tropical areas of the West Indies and the Pacific and Indian Oceans. Symptoms include gastroenteritis followed by neurological problems. (See Chapter 4 for further information on shellfish toxins.)
- Talk with your health-care provider about other advice regarding travel abroad.

Safe Water and Beverages

When traveling or camping in natural areas, we also need to take measures to assure the safety of our drinking water. Untreated water may harbor bacteria, parasites, or viruses. Mountain rivers, streams, and lakes often contain parasites such as giardia, cryptosporidium, or amoebas, as well as *E. coli* bacteria and viruses that can cause hepatitis. We can become infected by drinking or swimming in the water. When we travel, we have a few options concerning drinking water. First, on short trips or camping with a vehicle, we can carry our own water. When traveling in developing nations, it's best to totally avoid drinking the water. Instead, drink:

1. Beverages, such as tea and coffee, made with boiled water

2. Canned or bottled carbonated beverages such as sparkling waters and sodas since bacteria cannot exist when the level of carbon dioxide is high

3. Beer and wine

The only way to eradicate cryptosporidium is by boiling or filtering the water. Again, avoid drinks made with ice (or even food served on ice) since the ice can be contaminated.

In addition, there are three primary ways to purify water to make it safer—heat, chemicals, and filtration.

- **Boiled water.** At sea level, boiling water for 1 minute will kill bacteria and parasites. To kill viruses at altitudes above 6000 feet (about 2000 meters), boil the water for 3 minutes, or boil the water for 1 minute and also use chemical disinfectant.

- **Chemical treatment.** Using chemicals may be the simplest and the least expensive method, and yet it has drawbacks. Both iodine and chlorine have been used for this purpose. Of the two chemical methods, iodine is preferable, available in products such as Globaline, a form of crystalline iodine. One tablet can be added to a quart of water and will work in 10 minutes. Iodine can also be used in liquid solution—10 drops per quart. Let it sit for 30 minutes to kill the germs. However, it is important to note that iodine will not destroy cryptosporidium unless the water is allowed to sit for at least 15 hours. As for chlorine, the CDC states that "chlorine, in various forms, can also be used for chemical disinfection. However, its germicidal activity varies greatly with the . . . temperature and organic content of the water."[3] Overall, chemical treatment should be considered a last resort for water purification, but it is important to use when camping or traveling if other water purification resources are not available.

- **Filtration.** Filters designed for travel and camping are small portable units. Given the difficulty of boiling water at higher altitudes and the taste associated with chemical purification, filtration is a viable option. However, the filter used must be very fine — so select a unit that filters to 1 micron absolute. This will filter out most bacteria and parasites. Still, it will not remove viruses, which are typically smaller than 1 micron. In this event, the CDC recommends that, "To kill viruses, travelers using microstrainer filters should be advised to disinfect the water with iodine or chlorine after filtration."[4] When water cannot be boiled, the combination of filtration and disinfection appears to be a reasonable choice, since both giardia and cryptosporidium are larger than 1 micron — an example of why it's important to use filters labeled "1 micron absolute."

If you are wondering about the necessity of purifying your water, consider that in the United States alone, about 2 million people contract giardia each year, not only from city water systems, but also from state park water fountains and pristine mountain streams, so even backpackers in wilderness areas need to make provision for some type of water purification.

Air Travel

When you travel by air, you are essentially a captive audience, and may be exposed to many different types of infectious agents. This is especially true if you are sitting in front of or next to someone who is coughing and sneezing. You have no idea what you're being exposed to, and yet you can't just get up and walk away. Everyone who travels has experienced this.

For more than 20 years, airlines have been cutting costs by recirculating air within the cabin, rather than pumping in fresh air from outside as earlier planes did. Some research has suggested that recycled air does not increase the risk of contracting airborne illnesses such as colds and flu.[5] Yet other research found that about 19 percent of people traveling by plane contracted respiratory illness compared with a normal rate of these illnesses at about 7 percent.[6] Consequently, your best defense when flying is to boost your immune defenses right before, during, and after you travel with supplements containing transfer factors and other types of immune support. (Refer to the sidebar earlier in this chapter for further information on enhancing immunity during travel.)

Jet Lag

Several remedies are available to address jet lag. Of these, one of the most effective is melatonin, which can be used both to obtain additional sleep during travel and to "reset" your internal clock. Melatonin is a potent hormone, and so small doses are usually sufficient. Typically 3 to 6 mg are sufficient for jet lag. (See Resources for more information.) We mention jet lag here, because getting a good sleep is vital to strong immunity. While we sleep, key immune chemicals (including certain interleukins) rise in our blood, initiating a systemwide "housekeeping." This is one of the reasons that sleep has the ability to restore health. Managing jet lag also helps you maintain your resistance.

Environmental Factors

The environment can cause a wide range of health effects. Educate yourself well about the opportunities and potential exposures in the areas where you will be traveling. Environmental stress can leave you more vulnerable to other types of health problems.

- *High temperatures or heat and humidity* can lead to heat exhaustion if one becomes dehydrated. Increase your intake of nonalcoholic liquids, and monitor yourself (and your children) for the effects of excessive heat such as headache, dizziness, or hot, dry skin.
- *Extreme sunburn* can cause symptoms of physical illness. Use a hat and a sunscreen with a sun protection factor (SPF) of 15 or higher.
- *Exposure to excessive cold* can lead to hypothermia and even frostbite. Alcohol intake can dangerously intensify the effects of cold.
- *The effects of dust or air pollution* can cause fatigue and increase susceptibility to respiratory infections.
- *Reactions to toxic exposures* tend to be highly individual. Some countries have a policy of spraying airplane passenger cabins for insects (in areas of Latin America, the Caribbean, Australia, and the South Pacific). People with allergies or asthma may wish to inquire ahead about whether spraying (disinfection) will be performed on their flights. Further information can be obtained from the U.S. Department of Transportation on the web at www.ostpxweb.dot.gov/policy/safety/disin.htm.

Insect Repellent

Current recommendations on the use of repellents continue to favor the use of products that contain DEET (N,N-diethyl-meta-toluamide) as an active ingredient. To minimize exposure to toxicity, formulas are recommended which contain less than 10 to 35 percent DEET. For children, formulas of no more than 10 percent DEET are recommended and should be used sparingly on children ages 2 through 6. Again, be sure not to get repellent on a child's hands, and avoid contact with the child's eyes and mouth. Repellents should not be used on infants or toddlers under 2. Bed netting and a variety of insect repellents can be purchased in hardware and sporting goods stores. (For more information on minimizing exposure to insects and insect-borne illness, see Chapter 3 under Lyme disease.)

Hazards Due to Animals

Information on animal-related contagious illness can be reviewed in Chapter 11. You'll want to take a look at information on contagion in the environment, such as psittacosis carried by birds and transmitted in bird droppings. The content on rabies is also important since this virus is much more prevalent in developing nations than it is in industrial countries.

Swimming Precautions

Swimming in contaminated water can result in infections that affect the skin, eyes, or ears. Intestinal infections can also be contracted. Pools with chlorinated water are generally considered safe for swimming if chlorine levels are sufficiently high, although occasional rare problems are also associated with pool water. It is important to avoid beaches contaminated with human sewage or dog feces. The CDC also advises avoiding wading or swimming in freshwater streams, canals, and lakes infested with schistosoma (carried by snails) or contaminated with urine from animals carrying leptospira. Although schistosoma was once considered to be only found in the tropics, the disease has recently been identified in U.S. lakes as the cause of "swimmer's itch."

Cruise Ships

It's difficult to be sure which vaccines and preventive efforts are needed on a cruise since exposure onshore occurs for such brief periods of time. However, the CDC recommends that travelers on a cruise follow the prevention and vaccine recommendations that apply to each country visited. After consulting with a health-care provider, one may choose to modify the recommendations depending on the length of the visit ashore in any particular country.

In 2002 and 2003, more than 1500 cruise passengers contracted Norwalk virus or similar infections. The CDC provides an inspection program in cooperation with the cruise ship industry in which ships are periodically, randomly inspected and rated on sanitation. A score of 86 or higher indicates that the ship met acceptable standards at the time of inspection. Scores and inspection reports for each ship are available via the Internet at www.cdc.gov/nceh/vsp. Scores are also published every other week on a summary sheet, known as the "Green Sheet," distributed to travel-related services worldwide. (To obtain a copy by mail, see the information in the Resources section at the back of the book.)

Coping with Illness

When you travel, it's important to be prepared for the unexpected. You won't have access to your medicine cabinet, your kitchen cupboard, or the neighborhood pharmacy. We've suggested some basic supplements you can take when you're going to travel. You may find it helpful to make up a kit of nutrients and remedies, so if you come down with a minor illness, you can nip it in the bud. (See the Resources section for more information.) Your travel kit might include:

- Immune boosters.
- Antiviral and antibacterial herbs and remedies.
- Specific remedies for infections and other common problems.

Once You Return Home

Some of us do fine when we travel, but when we get home, we find that we have brought home a "souvenir" from our trip. Problems on returning home can range from digestive parasites to viral infections. In order to diagnose your problem, your doctor will want to know where you traveled (including stopovers), what you might have been exposed to and how long ago you were exposed, what season of the year it was, and what vaccinations you have had.[7]

Fever

The presence of a fever can reflect any of a great number of infectious illnesses. World travel broadens the list of possible exposures and increases the careful detective work required of your physician to diagnose a possible problem. The incubation period and source of exposure help to narrow the problem. For example, among travelers returning from the tropics with fever symptoms, the most frequent causes of illness include malaria, enteric fever (especially typhoid or paratyphoid fever), hepatitis A, and dengue. Symptoms should be checked out and monitored carefully. Sicknesses such as malaria and enteric fever may begin simply as a fever, but they can result in life-threatening complications. Table 12.2 lists conditions most often associated with fever.

Table 12.2   Possible Origins of Fever in Returning Travelers

Incubation period

Less than 10 days	10 to 21 days	More than 21 days	Variable
• Dengue	• Malaria	• Malaria	• Drug fever
• Enteric fever	• Enteric fever	• Hepatitis A to E	
• Typhus	• Typhus	• Brucellosis	
• Yellow fever	• Hepatitis A and E	• Visceral leishmaniasis	
• Legionnaires' disease	• Leptospirosis	• Rabies	
• Relapsing fever	• African trypanosomiasis	• Acute schistosomiasis	
• Plague	• Chagas' disease	• Tuberculosis	
• Mosquitoborne or tickborne encephalitis	• Q fever	• Extraintestinal amoebiasis	
	• Relapsing fever	• Melioidosis	
• Bacterial sepsis	• Encephalitis	• Filariasis	
• Influenza	• Brucellosis	• Acute HIV infection	
	• Melioidosis		

SOURCE: Reproduced with the permission of Health Press Limited from A. J. Pollard and D. R. Murdoch. *Fast Facts—Travel Medicine*. Oxford: Health Press, 2001.

Diarrhea

This is not an uncommon symptom, and it's most often caused by parasites or bacteria. Typically, traveler's diarrhea lasts less than a week. Diarrhea that persists longer than 4 weeks is considered a chronic condition and can be due to bacteria, protozoa, helminths (worms), or other causes. Many of the same bad bugs that cause food poisoning at home are responsible for digestive upsets that occur when traveling, including types of *E. coli*, salmonella, shigella, campylobacter, and cholera-related illness (vibrio species) (see Table 12.3). The CDC indicates that a number of studies implicated rotaviruses in as many as one-third of the cases of traveler's diarrhea evaluated. The CDC also points out the possibility of parasitic infection, which must be identified by lab testing, and indicates that "the likelihood of

---

Table 12.3 Possible Causes of Diarrhea in the Returning Traveler

Bacteria	**Helminths**
• Campylobacter	• Schistosoma
• Shigellosis	• Hookworm
• *Clostridium difficile*	• Strongyloides
• Other types of acute bacterial diarrhea	

Protozoa	**Noninfectious causes**
• Giardia	• Medications
• Amoebas (*E. histolytica*)	• Irritable bowel syndrome
• Cryptosporidium	• Deficiency of digestive enzymes
• Cyclospora	

SOURCE: Reproduced with the permission of Health Press Limited from A. J. Pollard and, D. R. Murdoch. *Fast Facts—Travel Medicine*. Oxford: Health Press, 2001.

a parasitic [infection] is higher when diarrheal illness is prolonged. *E. histolytica* [amoebas] should be considered when the patient has dysentery or invasive diarrhea (bloody stools)."[8] Both diarrhea and constipation should be taken seriously. It is important to note that these conditions can be difficult to diagnose, and their role in human illness is not fully appreciated. Be sure to follow up on symptoms that persist and get them resolved. An integrative approach can be helpful in dealing with the types of digestive disorders that develop when traveling.

Increased Immune activity

An elevated total white blood count can show increased activity of the immune system and the likely presence of infection. When blood tests show an elevated eosinophile level (a component of the white blood cell count) this points to the presence of a parasitic infection or an allergic condition (see Table 12.4). Elevated eosinophils are also associated with other types of infection. In addition, other components of the white count may also be

---

Table 12.4   Causes of Increased Immune Activity (Eosinophils)

Parasitic causes	Nonparasitic causes
• Nematodes including ascaris, hookworm, strongyloides, filaria, toxacara, trichinosis	• Allergies, including dermatitis and asthma
• Trematodes, including schistosoma	• Reactions to drugs ranging from antibiotics and nonsteroidal anti-inflammatory drugs to aspirin
• Others	

SOURCE: Reproduced with the permission of Health Press Limited from A. J. Pollard and D. R Murdoch. *Fast Facts—Travel Medicine*. Oxford: Health Press, 2001.

elevated (such as neutrophils or lymphocytes). These are also indicators of increased immune activity and other types of infections as well.

Travel Resources

If you plan to travel overseas, check with the embassy or consulate of the countries you will be visiting, as well as their embassy in the United States, for health tips, required vaccinations, and possible concerns. The U.S. consulate often has a list of recommended doctors, dentists, and hospitals in specific countries. At the back of this book, the Resources section includes a bibliography of useful books on travel and travel health.

13

SARS:
Coping with an
Emerging Epidemic

WHEN SARS IS JUST A MEMORY, it is our hope that the information in this chapter will not be forgotten, because, unfortunately,
there is no question that there will continue to be new and
emerging epidemics in the future. Hopefully, these preventive
strategies will still be a part of your life—steps you take on a daily
basis. However, there are additional perspectives here that you
might want to keep for reference and revisit at the time of the
next emerging infection or epidemic.

The entire globe is now closely linked through international travel and trade. An epidemic anywhere in the world is
only one plane ride away. New forms of infectious illness also
emerge as we disrupt ancient ecosystems across the planet—for
example, the rain forests in South America, Africa, New Guinea,
and Madagascar. Rain forests contain not only exotic plants and
animals but also exotic microbes such as the Ebola virus.

SARS Overview

1. Profiling the Germ

We'll provide an overview of the SARS virus here, but you can apply this same game plan to any form of contagion or infection, from West Nile virus to the flu. You can train yourself to think in terms of:

- **What type of microbe is it?** Is it bacteria, virus, fungus, parasite, or some other organism?
- **How is it transmitted?** Is it focused in a certain geographic area or a particular environment. (Lyme is harbored by woodland ticks, whereas West Nile virus is mosquito-borne, so it tends to be more prevalent around water or areas where water pools.)
- **How does this relate to you and your lifestyle?** Do you have a job that exposes you to a great many people? Do you go hiking or backpacking? Which germs do you need to guard against?

2. Assessing the Seriousness of the Situation

Any situation that involves loss of life is serious. But before we panic, it's important to remember that *fear* can depress the immune system, decreasing our resistance to infection. To date, SARS is actually less deadly than the flu, which kills more than 20,000 people each year in the United States alone. At the time of this writing there are about 8000 reported cases of SARS worldwide and more than 650 reported deaths.[1] This is a fatality rate of about 8 percent.

Our public health service, using telecommunications and technology, has been able to launch into full operation with breathtaking speed. The SARS virus was identified only 3 *weeks* after the potential of an epidemic was recognized. The scale of our mass media is also unprecedented, which means that we all have access to an enormous amount of information. The downside is that we get media exposure to every detail of the epidemic. This tends to amplify our perception of the threat, with the potential to keep us in a state of constant tension. So one strategy for dealing with this is to minimize information overload.

You don't want to be in fear, because fear can get in the way of living fully in the present. That can take away your appreciation for life and the richness of experience from moment to moment. Fear can also depress your immunity, just as any form of stress can. On the other hand, you don't want to be unrealistic. If you are, you may be tempted to falsely assume that there are no risks, and, as a result, you might not alter your behavior in an appropriate way. It's important to use smart preventive strategies to protect yourself.

3. Developing Preventive Strategies

You can look at any epidemic in terms of focused prevention. Public health authorities have their role, and we encourage you to play your part as well. What can you do to strengthen your body against this particular germ?

SARS Overview *(Continued)*

- **Healthy lifestyle.** The efforts you make on a daily basis to stay healthy can affect your body's ability to fight an infection.
- **Nutrients and herbs.** Taking these things helps fight viruses and bacteria and boosts the immune system.
- **Targeted prevention.** Strengthen the organs most affected by the germ, such as the lungs in the case of SARS.
- **Minimize exposure.** It's wise to avoid areas where there is a known epidemic.

The SARS Virus

Fact

SARS—Severe Acute Respiratory Syndrome—is a form of "atypical pneumonia" caused by a virus. The first cases occurred in November 2002 in southern China. The epidemic was first widely reported in March 2003, and the virus was identified 3 weeks later.

Germ

- **A coronavirus.** SARS is caused by an aggressive new strain of the coronavirus, a group of viruses that have a halo or crownlike (corona) appearance when viewed under a microscope. This class of viruses includes the microbe that causes the common cold in about one-third of all cases. Infections due to coronaviruses can trigger much more severe symptoms in animals, including respiratory, intestinal, liver, and neurological diseases. The SARS virus apparently began as some form of animal virus and then "jumped species."[2] The aggressiveness of some coronaviruses in animals may explain the virulence of this new, more threatening form of the virus.

At first, researchers explored the possibility that the SARS virus might have mutated from the Hong Kong bird flu of 1997, which resurfaced in 1999. Working almost around the clock, researchers eventually identified this new virus using various types of testing, including evaluations of genetic material (PCR testing) and of immune markers (antibodies), as well as observation with high-powered electron microscopes.

Coronaviruses are among the viruses that have an extra outer shell, or envelope, so they are described as "enveloped." Enveloped viruses require close contact for transmission. The virus forms the envelope from the host cell's membrane, which can result in immune reactions such as inflammation, swelling, or autoimmune reactions. This may be one of the factors that contributes to the severity of the response in SARS.

- **Possible coinfections.** The World Health Organization (WHO) reports that in Hong Kong, there is a pattern of transmission "different from what is being seen in the vast majority of other SARS outbreaks."[3] There is the suspicion that some of the coronavirus infections occur in conjunction with another virus (paramyxovirus). This would explain why some of those with the virus transmit the illness to many people, while others who are infected do not appear to be very contagious.[4] A number of other puzzling patterns have emerged. For example, researchers wonder why one of the early victims of SARS was not contagious to his four adult children, who were living in his household, though he did transmit the virus to other people he encountered outside the home.[5] In addition, SARS has also been linked to a rare airborne form of chlamydia bacteria. This raises the question of whether the infection is caused by one virus or bacteria and made more deadly by another.[6] Currently, these issues and others are still under investigation by the CDC and the WHO.

Geography

- **Location.** SARS is believed to have originated in southern China, and was transmitted to Hong Kong, Canada, Singapore, and Vietnam. By late May 2003, approximately 8000 cases of SARS had been reported, with more than 650 deaths (approximately 8 percent of those infected).

SARS has also "continued to go global, affecting more than 28 countries, as infected individuals jetted from hot zones to other parts of the world, passing along their unwelcome baggage through sneezes and coughs."[7] SARS has also been reported in Australia, Britain, Canada, France, Japan, the United States, and Taiwan. In some cases, the virus appears to grow weaker as it is replicated over and over.

- **Environmental factors.** The SARS virus emerged in one of the rural provinces located south of Hong Kong. Intensive farming methods that are practiced in this area (and in many other areas worldwide) in effect cluster many animals together, creating conditions that allow new diseases to spread rapidly. Pigs are frequently a vector, because they can be infected by human viruses as well as by pathogens from animals such as rodents and fowl. As a result, pigs provide a "host environment" in which microbes can mutate and jump from animal species to humans.[8]

Symptoms

- **Symptoms.** SARS often begins with a fever of 100.4°or higher. Among those who have contracted SARS, almost 100 percent have had fever, chills, and fatigue. Less than half actually develop a cough or a sore throat. In the majority of cases, the symptoms begin as severe headache, dizziness, and aching muscles, with a continual fever. After 2 to 7 days, patients often develop a dry cough and may progress to difficulty with breathing.[9] In some cases, oxygen levels drop rapidly and 10 to 20 percent of patients require ventilator support.

If you have any of these flu-like symptoms and are experiencing difficulty breathing, it's important to see your doctor or go to an emergency room immediately.

- **Airborne transmission.** The virus is spread through close personal contact, by droplet transmission, and by coughs or sneezes. It also appears to be conveyed by touch, so handwashing is important. There is concern that it may also have spread in Hong Kong through ventilation systems, waterborne transmission in sewage, or by a vector such as the cockroach. It is possible that the virus is also transmitted by adhering to surfaces, where it is believed to survive for a few hours.
- **Who is at risk?** Most cases of SARS occur among people who have had direct close contact with an

infected person—someone in the household or a health-care worker. Once contracted, its effects are generally more harmful in the elderly or those with preexisting medical conditions.

- **Incubation period.** The virus typically has a 3 to 5 day incubation period, although symptoms may appear within 2 days. Public health officials have asked those who have been exposed to isolate themselves for a full 10 days before assuming they do not have SARS.

- **Atypical pneumonia.** SARS can trigger an "inflammatory storm" as the immune system attempts to fight off the virus, causing the lung tissue to swell. In 10 to 20 percent of cases, patients need to be on a ventilator. In severe cases, suffocation can result due to the inflammation and swelling in the lungs.

Minimizing Exposure

- **This particular virus is airborne.** The SARS virus is transmitted by close contact and in crowded places. If you or a member of your family has SARS, the CDC suggests that you wear a mask, which can be purchased in a medical supply store. The most common type of mask is one that filters out any particle larger than 1 micron. However, it's important to remember that all viruses, including SARS, are far smaller than 1 micron. This means that these masks will screen out contamination such as mucus and droplets transmitted by a cough or a sneeze. However, they do not filter out airborne viruses. Health-care professionals will want to use the N-95 respirator.

- **It is transmitted by touch and may also adhere to surfaces.** You can minimize surface transmission of the virus by periodically wiping surfaces you touch with alcohol or alcohol wipes. This approach was found successful in removing germs from doctors' pagers. It may also be helpful to clean your computer keyboard and your phone when you arrive at work each morning. If someone in the home has SARS, don't share silverware, towels, or bedding until they have been washed with soap and hot water. Clean surfaces that have been contaminated by body fluids (sweat, saliva, mucus, vomit, or urine) with a household disinfectant and disposable gloves. All cleaning materials and gloves should be discarded after each use.

Frequent handwashing is one of the most important things you can do — and be sure to wash your hands before you eat. You may want to carry sanitizing towelettes if you don't have access to soap and water at work or at school. (Parents: Note that in many public schools, soap is no longer available. It is advisable to have your children carry soap in their backpacks, just as you might when you go to the gym or when you travel. Another option is to have them use some form of nonalcohol hand sanitizers. Two studies on handwashing found an average 50 percent decrease in illness among children who washed their hands before meals.[10,11]

- **Respect travel advisories.** More than two-thirds of the cases have occurred in mainland China and Hong Kong. The WHO initially issued an alert, advising travelers to postpone nonessential trips to Hong Kong and Gaungdong province, as well as geographic areas outside China.

- **Isolation and quarantine.** Those who have been exposed to the SARS virus have been asked to voluntarily isolate themselves by staying home for 10 days. The U.S. government has put measures in place that enable it to detain people in quarantine. Isolation is intended to separate those who have contracted an illness from those who are healthy in order to prevent the spread of disease. A *contact* is someone with symptoms who has had close contact during the preceding 10 days with a person who is a suspected or probable case of SARS. A *close contact* is a person who has cared for, lived with, or had direct contact with respiratory secretions or body fluids of a suspected or probable case of SARS. In hospitals, isolation protocols for SARS are observed so that the virus will not spread to other patients. One strategy for controlling the spread of the infection is to identify highly infectious people, termed "super-spreaders." Health officials have also tried to minimize the spread of SARS by encouraging people with symptoms of the infection to avoid air travel.

In Hong Kong and Singapore, where the outbreak began, many schools were closed. Air travel slowed—18 percent of Hong Kong's flights were canceled. In Canada, two hospitals were closed in response to the epidemic, and 1800 employees were sent home. In Singapore, 1700 people exposed to the SARS virus were confined to their homes.

Preventive Strategies

Currently there is no known form of treatment that specifically addresses the SARS virus. This makes prevention all the more important. The most effective approach works on several levels at once:

- **Level 1—Immune Prevention.** The first, most basic level of prevention involves supporting the immune system. For example, are you getting enough vitamin A and zinc, which are *essential* to immune activity? Your body literally can't mount an effective attack without these nutrients. When your immune system is well maintained, then if you do come in contact with this virus (or any other), your body provides a less-hospitable environment. If the virus does gain access, it is more likely to be kept in check by your immune system. As a result, the virus is less likely to replicate and less likely to do damage.

- **Level 2 — Microbe Prevention.** SARS is caused by a virus, and there are specific nutrients and herbs you can take that have antiviral activity. You can apply this same protocol at a later time with other viruses. In other situations, you might be dealing with a bacteria or a fungus, so you would use other antimicrobial strategies, both conventional and alternative, depending on the particular germ you're dealing with.
- **Level 3 — Targeted Prevention.** SARS infections are a form of atypical pneumonia. When you are thinking preventively in this scenario, this means protecting and strengthening the lungs. In Chinese medicine, the lungs are considered to be the defensive armor of the body (called the *Wei Qi*). In other words, the lungs are your first line of defense against airborne exposure. (See also Chapter 7.)

Nip Infections in the Bud

This does not mean self-treating a serious illness, such as SARS. At the first sign of a minor cold or the flu, take steps to resolve the illness as quickly as possible. This will keep your lungs, ears, nose, and throat as healthy as possible, keeping your mucus membranes free of infection. This also helps to maintain your immune defenses. Then if you are exposed to a more ferocious germ, your immune system will still be able to provide a strong defense. In that case, you may not catch it, or, if you do, you are more likely to be one of the 92 percent who survive it. The stronger your immunity, the less of an effect an infection will have on your body—by definition, you will be better able to fight it off.

Treatment

There are different approaches to treating the SARS virus. (See Table 13.1.)

Conventional Treatment

Testing is being done to determine the most effective antiviral medication. At the time of this writing, there is currently no known specific treatment for SARS. In mainstream medicine, the primary therapy for SARS infections is a broad spectrum ("shotgun") approach consisting of an intravenous cocktail of antiviral and antibiotic medications. Ribavirin is an antiviral given in combination with antibacterials such as Rocephin and Zithromax in case there is a secondary infection. Steroids are included in the IV to minimize inflammation, particularly the swelling in the lung membranes, which can result in suffocation. Additionally, ventilation is required if the patient's oxygen levels drop below a certain level.

A simple test is available that enables your physician to monitor your oxygen level if you have respiratory symptoms and he or she suspects you may have SARS or any other form of

Table 13.1 SARS Treatment Strategies

Therapies	How They Work	Prevention	Early Stage of Any Viral Illness	Integrative Treatment
Conventional Medication				
Ribavirin Rocephin Zithromax	Antivirals and antibacterials			Given intravenously
Immune Boosters				
Transfer Factor	Antiviral, immune-stimulating peptides	1 cap–3x/ per day	2 caps–3x/ per day	3 to 4 caps–3x/ per day
Transfer Factor Plus	Includes extracts of immune-enhancing Chinese mushrooms	1 cap per day	1 cap–2x/ per day	2 caps–2–3x/ per day
Vitamin Therapy				
Multivitamin	Broad nutritional support	Use on an ongoing basis	Use on an ongoing basis	Use on an ongoing basis
Vitamin C	Antiviral, immune-stimulating	1000 mg,, 1 to 2x/per day	1000 mg,, 3 to 4x/per day	2000 mg, 2 to 3x/per day
Vitamin A	Helps fight infection, heals mucosal tissue	Contained in multivitamin	25,000 iu/per drop or cap 1 to 2x/per day for 5 days only	Discuss higher doses with your integrative physician

Continued on next page

285

Table 13.1 *(continued)*

Therapies	How They Work	Prevention	Early Stage of Any Viral Illness	Integrative Treatment
Omega 3 Essential Fatty Acids	Support the immune system	1 gel cap–3x/ per day	2 gel caps–3x/ per day	3 gel caps–3x/ per day
Herbs				
Olive leaf extract, echinacae, garlic, ginger, licorice	Anti-inflammatory and antiviral	Dose varies with form and concentration of the herbs.		
Homeopathy	Antiviral		GrippHeel–1 cap every 2 hours for the first day, then 1 cap 3x/per day for 5 to 7 days	
Chinese Herbal Formulas				
Isatis Gold	Treats viral and bacterial infection		3 tabs–3x/per day (for 7 to 10 days)	
Astra 8	Adaptogen–helps the body adapt to stress, immune enhancer, strengthens lungs	2 tabs–3x/ per day (can be taken continuously)	2 tabs–3x/ per day (can be taken continuously)	

286

Continued on next page

Table 13.1 *(continued)*

Therapies	How They Work	Prevention	Early Stage of Any Viral Illness	Integrative Treatment
Individual Chinese Antivirals Astragalus, forsythia and honeysuckle, ganoderma mushroom, isatis, or schizandra	Immune-enhancing and/or antiviral activity	Dose varies depending on product.		
Probiotics Acidophilas, bifidus, and saccharomyces boulardii	Promotes GI health, prevents fungal overgrowth	1 cap—1x/ per day (taken daily)	1 cap—1x/ per day (taken daily)	1 cap—2 to 3x/ per day when taking antibiotics

287

pneumonia. This noninvasive test, pulse oximetry, is available in emergency rooms and most health-care facilities. The test can show decreasing oxygen levels in the blood, helpful in determining if the symptoms reflect simply a respiratory infection or if they are causing damage to your lungs.

Innovative Treatment

One of the treatments in Hong Kong that has resulted in improved survival has been the use of blood products (containing serum from recovered SARS patients), which transmit immune protective factors to patients with active disease.[12] (Serum injections were also used successfully against the Ebola virus.) The fact that doctors are able to obtain these factors from the blood of recovering patients means these patients are successfully producing antibodies—"artillery" made by the immune system to fight the virus. Such innovative treatments are being used overseas. They also highlight the tremendous therapeutic potential of therapies that support the immune defenses.

Immune-Supportive Therapies

Using an immune-based approach holds promise for the development of future therapies for SARS and other viruses. Potential therapies focused on immune support include vaccines (preventive), gamma globulin (postinfection), and transfer factors (preventive and postinfection). There is currently an enormous amount of research on these immune-based approaches.

Therapies that transmit immune-protective factors are of particular value in the treatment of an illness for which there is no specific treatment (no magic bullet), and also relevant in situations in which the microbial threat is of unknown origin.

Strong immunity is ultimately the basis for fighting any infection. Even with the use of antibiotics, the goal is to lower the levels of bacteria so that the immune system can destroy any harmful bacteria that remain, as well as postinfectious debris. Because the immune system is the common denominator in all illness, immune therapies have universal relevance.

The immune system is affected by a broad range of factors—genetic tendencies, immune compromise, and lifestyle practices that tend to lower immune function, as well as hidden infections that can be a drain on immunity. It is possible that some people are seriously affected by SARS due to this constellation of factors. For example, the individual response to the enveloped virus may also be an added factor. The inflammatory crisis that can result is a major cause of the fatalities.

Considering susceptibility from the perspective of immune health, we look at these factors on a continuum and evaluate the individual's ability to resist illness. The health of the immune system also determines the severity of inflammatory or autoimmune reactions in the presence of an infection. Why do some some people develop an "inflammatory storm" while others go unscathed? These aspects of immunity may contribute to the patient's individual response, but at the time of this writing, many questions wait to be answered through future research regarding immune function.

Using Integrative Medicine

If you have any symptoms of SARS, or suspect a SARS infection, see a doctor immediately. To date, there is no known specific antiviral treatment for SARS infections. If you want to use integrative medicine, it is important to have an integrative physician on your medical team, which might also consist of your family physician or internist, an infectious disease specialist, pulmonary specialist, or critical care specialist, and so on.

Resources

You can obtain additional information and links regarding SARS, emerging infections, and finding an integrative physician by visiting our web site at www.germsurvivalguide.com. Information on this outbreak can be obtained on the web site of the CDC at www.cdc.gov and from the World Health Organization at www.who.int.

14

Germ Warfare— What You Can Do to Protect Your Family

UNTIL THE aftermath of September 11, 2001, it's a pretty safe bet to say that the majority of us hadn't given much thought to anthrax, that most people believed smallpox was a disease they would never have to encounter again, that the plague was confined to the pages of history books, that botulinum toxin came from spoiled food in a can, and that tularemia was—well, had anyone even ever heard of it?

Our world has changed, and so has the way we talk about it. These once foreign or uncommon words are now becoming a part of everyday vocabulary. They are in newspapers and magazines; they come to us over the TV and radio. And whenever these words cross our paths, they are linked with one chilling idea: bioterrorism.

While we can see and thus more readily appreciate the destruction and terror associated with the use of bullets, tanks, and bombs, the instruments of germ warfare are invisible to the naked eye. Although many different generations have grappled with potential public health crises from invisible enemies, from smallpox and polio in the early twentieth century to herpes, HIV, and hepatitis C in the 1980s and 1990s, the unseen enemy we are now facing is different. While, for the most part, the afore-mentioned health crises cropped up naturally, the ones we now face are initiated with malicious intent by groups, individuals, or other entities for the purpose of spreading terror and death.

But we don't have to let the terrorists win. Is the threat of serious illness and death from these "new" bioterrorism agents any worse than that from the bacterial and viral infections with which we are now familiar, like the flu or pneumonia? Only if we let them be. We do have tools to prevent, fight, and treat bioterrorism agents. These tools address not only our physical health but our emotional, mental, and spiritual well-being as well. This chapter explains each of the biological threats and what you can do to protect yourself and your family.

The Centers for Disease Control and Prevention,[1] the Johns Hopkins Center for Civilian Biodefense,[2] the Mayo Clinic,[3] and other esteemed institutions have identified the most likely (and current) weapons of bioterrorism. They fall into three major categories (the first two of which are biological):

- **Bacteriological.** Anthrax, plague, tularemia, and botulinum toxin
- **Viral.** Smallpox
- **Chemical.** Nerve gases, including mustard gas, chlorine, sarin, hydrogen cyanide, and phosgene

Germ Warfare

It would be convenient if each of these biological threats could be prevented or treated by simply taking an antibiotic. How-ever, that isn't the case. The agents in each of these categories work on the body in different ways and are also treated differently medically. Before we get into a discussion of how each of us can combat bioterrorism, it's helpful to understand what we're dealing with. By knowing your enemy, you will be better able to overcome it. We're going to look at each of the biological agents in all three categories, with special emphasis on those in the bacteriological and viral groups.

Anthrax

If you're involved in agriculture or raising farm animals, you may have heard about anthrax before the recent crisis. Anthrax, a disease that usually affects livestock, is caused by spore-forming bacteria called *Bacillus anthracis*, derived from the Greek word for coal, *anthrakis*, because the disease causes black, coal-like skin lesions. These bacteria usually live in soil in spores that are odorless, tasteless, and invisible to the unaided eye. Anthrax spores are so small, in fact, that you could put millions of them into a thimble. Yet it takes an amount only as small as a speck of dust to make someone ill.

Anthrax spores germinate when they enter a host, such as a cow or human, because the host provides the right environment—amino acids and glucose (sugar), for example, found in blood and tissues. The spores change into the anthrax bacteria, which then produce a deadly toxin. We've discussed the transmission of germs. Anthrax can enter the body in three different ways:

- **Through the skin.** Cutaneous anthrax is caused by spores that enter a break in the skin. The resulting infection at first looks like an insect bite, but within a few days it develops into an open lesion with a black center. If untreated, it kills one in five infected people.

- **Through inhalation.** Inhalation anthrax occurs when the spores are breathed into the lungs. About 12 hours after exposure, symptoms that resemble a mild cold or flu (e.g., fatigue, dry cough, low-grade fever) appear. After several days, however, the infection causes a high fever, shock, and pneumonia. About 90 percent of people who get inhalation anthrax die.
- **Through food.** Intestinal anthrax develops when people eat meat from an infected animal. This form of anthrax causes inflammation of the intestines, loss of appetite, vomiting of blood, and severe diarrhea. Between 25 and 60 percent of those untreated patients die.

All three forms of anthrax are treatable with antibiotics if treatment is begun as soon as symptoms are evident (see Table 14.1). None of the forms are contagious. You can be exposed to anthrax and not become infected, since whether or not you get the disease depends on the degree of exposure and the virulence of the strain to which you were exposed. Although anthrax has been spread in a powder form through the mail, experts say that the technology does not exist to distribute it from a crop-dusting plane or from the head of a missile.

Smallpox

Of the five biological weapons we discuss, smallpox is the only virus. Most people believed that smallpox was wiped off the face of the earth in the late 1970s, but in reality, stocks of the virus exist in at least two World Health Organization labs. It's unknown whether terrorists have supplies of their own.

The variola virus causes smallpox. The virus is easily transmitted through the air, which means that an aerosol

Table 14.1 Combating Bioterrorism: A Personal Plan

Disease	Anthrax	Smallpox	Plague	Tularemia	Botulism
Agent	Bacteria	Virus	Bacteria	Bacteria	Toxin
Means of Infection	Inhalation Skin Contact Ingestion	Person-to-person	Inhalation	Inhalation Ingestion in food or water	Inhalation Ingestion in food
Incubation	1 to 42 days	7 to 14 days	2 to 3 days	2 to 10 days	2 hours to 8 days
Potential to Cause Illness	90% on inhalation	30% of those not vaccinated	100% without treatment	5 to 10%	5 to 60% in those vaccinated
Vaccine	Vaccine for military use only. Long-term side effects	Administer within 3 days of contact	Available, but not effective against inhaled strain	Available	Antitoxin vaccined can be used once infected
Symptoms	Flu-like symptoms: fever, cough, weakness, pneumonia	Flu-like symptoms: fever, rash, headache, pneumonia	Cough, fever, pneumonia, bleeding	Fever, chills, swollen lymph glands, pneumonia	Headache, vomiting, diarrhea, difficulty swallowing or speaking
Conventional Treatment	Doxycycline for 60 days or Cipro for 60 days	Cidofovir	Tetracycline, doxycycline, cipro, or streptomycin for 7 days	Doxycycline for 14 days or streptomycin for 11 to 14 days	Antitoxin vaccine, temporary respirator support until toxin dissipates

Continued on next page

295

Table 14.1 (continued)

An Integrative Approach—in *addition* to the above precautions and treatments

Disease	Anthrax	Smallpox	Plague	Tularemia
Specific Immune Support	• Astragalus	• IP-6 • Vitamin C, 2,000 mg, 3x day	• Astragalus	• Antioxidant support
Homeopathics		• Variolinum for 2 weeks • Vaccination for 1 week following vaccine		• Lymphomyosot, to help minimize edema and flu-like symptoms
Basic Support	• A high-potency, balanced multivitamin with antioxidants and B vitamins • Probiotic supplement with aciodophilus, bifidus, and s. boulardii whenever antibiotics are taken • Milk thistle to protect liver			
General Immune Support	• Vitamin A • Nutritional formula for immune support			
Nutrients and Herbal Support	• Lactoferrin for viral-, bacterial-, or toxin-related infection • Antimicrobials such as oil of oregano, olive leaf extract, andrographis, Resist, Citricidal			

296

release over a populated area would result in a high percentage of smallpox cases. The virus can also be transmitted person-to-person, and only a very small amount is needed for people to become infected.

People can be exposed to smallpox but not develop symptoms for 12 to 14 days, the average incubation period. After the incubation period, infected individuals experience fatigue, high fever, and body aches, followed by a rash. The disease gets its name from these pocks—small, pus-filled, round blisters that are embedded in the skin. Some patients have delirium and severe abdominal pain. The rash typically first appears inside the mouth and on the face and forearms. It then spreads to the trunk and legs. After 8 or 9 days, crusts begin to form. Once the scabs fall off, pitted scars eventually form.

Smallpox can be fatal within weeks; however, not everyone who gets the disease dies. Smallpox is fatal in about 30 percent of cases. In nonfatal cases, the disease runs its course in about 4 weeks. Researchers have never discovered an effective treatment for smallpox, but there is a vaccine and there are remedies you can take to counteract its side effects. In 1972, vaccinations for smallpox were stopped in the United States, and it is believed that anyone who had previously received the vaccine no longer has immunity.

Plague

As kids we learned about the Black Plague, or Black Death, in grade school, and then we didn't think about it again. After all, it could never affect us, right?

Plague, a disease caused by the bacteria *Yersinia pestis*, still exists, although just a few cases break out around the world each year. However, in the 1950s and 1960s, the biological weapons programs in both the United States and the Soviet Union developed techniques to aerosolize plague particles, which means both nations could release a highly deadly and contagious form of pneumonic plague. Terrorists could also have this ability.

An outbreak of plague following a biological attack would behave differently from one that occurred naturally. The severity and extent of the attack would depend on factors such as the amount of particles released, their potency, the weather conditions, and the way the particles were disseminated. Experts believe that the first cases would appear about 1 to 2 days after the aerosol exposure and that the incubation period would be 1 to 6 days. Because there is no way to detect an aerosol release of plague bacteria, the first sign of a bioterrorist attack would probably be sudden reports of people having severe symptoms. Those symptoms include fever with cough and difficulty breathing, sometimes with watery, bloody, or purulent (containing pus) sputum. Nausea, vomiting, abdominal pain, and diarrhea may be present as well. The clinical signs are similar to those of rapidly progressive pneumonia. Plague infections are treatable with antibiotics. (Also see Table 14.1.)

Tularemia

Tularemia—not exactly a household word, but it could be. Considered to be a dangerous potential biological weapon, tularemia is caused by a hardy bacterium called *Francisella tularensis*. The organism is extremely infectious and easy to disseminate, and can cause a great number of people to become ill or die.

The U.S. military stockpiled tularemia bacteria until the late 1960s and then destroyed it in the early 1970s. The Soviet Union continued to produce antibiotic- and vaccine-resistant strains until the early 1990s. The bacteria can be spread by inhalation of airborne bacteria; by direct contact with or ingestion of contaminated water, food, soil, or animal tissues; or through bites from infected animals. The good news: It does not appear to be contagious among people.

According to a World Health Organization expert committee, *F. tularensis* dispersed through the air (aerosol) over a populated area would cause a sudden large number of cases of fever beginning 3 to 5 days after the attack (incubation range, 1 to 14 days). Over the next few days and weeks, other symptoms would develop, such as headache, chills, weakness, and enlarged, tender lymph nodes. Without antibiotic treatment, the disease could progress to pneumonia, respiratory failure, shock, and death.

Botulism

Most of us have seen a "pregnant" can of food—one that has puffed out at either end because of the spoiled food inside. Eating such contaminated food will give you a case of botulism, a potentially deadly condition caused by botulinum toxin. Botulinum toxin also has a good side: It can be used to treat specific nerve conditions, such as crossed eyes, and it can be used to help eliminate facial wrinkles. Obviously, in this form it is given only under the strict supervision of a physician.

But botulinum toxin is also a biological weapon, and it is the single most poisonous substance known. Seven different types of the toxin exist, and all are made by a bacterium called *Clostridium botulinum*. Botulism results when the toxin is absorbed by the gut, in the lungs, or through a wound. The toxin cannot penetrate intact skin. If botulinum toxin were used as a biological weapon, it would likely be released through food contamination. No cases of waterborne botulism have ever been reported, probably because the toxin is easily neutralized by common water treatment methods.

If there were a deliberate food-borne release of botulinum toxin, it could be detected in several ways: (1) a large number of cases reported at once, (2) cases showing the same toxin type (remember, there are seven strains), (3) multiple simultaneous outbreaks of botulism without a common source, and (4) cases that shared a common geographic area but did not have a common food exposure.

The incubation period for food-borne and airborne botulism can range from 2 hours to 8 days after the contaminated substance has been ingested, although the average time is 12 to 72 hours. Once in the body, the toxin typically causes nausea, vomiting, diarrhea, and stomach cramps, followed by difficulty speaking, blurred or double vision, dry mouth, drooping eyelids, and trouble swallowing. Individuals may experience muscle weakness and paralysis that starts at the top of the body and moves down. The disease can kill by paralyzing the breathing muscles.

The severity of symptoms can vary, depending on the amount of toxin absorbed. It can take several weeks or months to recover from paralysis, because the body needs to replace damaged motor nerve endings. Treatment is available for botulism, and most people recover with prompt attention.

Stress and Fear: Controllable Biological Weapons

Terrorists may attempt to strike fear into our hearts, minds, and souls, but we need to remember what President Franklin Roosevelt said so many decades ago: *The only thing we have to fear is fear itself.* Therefore, we have a choice: We can allow the terrorists to succeed by letting fear and stress take over our lives, thus allowing these emotions to become the ultimate biological weapon; or we can choose to take control of our response to fear and stress. We do have the power to decide how we will respond to bioterrorism.

How we choose to respond is critical to our overall health, because the body will react to how we perceive fearful and stressful situations. Although stress affects different systems in the body—the nervous, immune, and endocrine systems—all these systems are in constant communication with each other. Thus the responses generated by any one of them impacts the others.

Psychoneuroimmunology is the study of the interrelationship between the nervous, immune, and endocrine systems. These three systems communicate with each other via special biochemical messengers: neurotransmitters in the nervous system, hormones in the endocrine system, and cytokines in the immune system. We know this interaction occurs because, for example, there are receptors for neurotransmitters on immune cells and there are receptors for cytokines on certain nerve cells. So when stress is added to the picture, it's intriguing to see how these three systems interact.

The Nervous System

The central nervous system (the brain and spinal cord) includes the autonomic nervous system, which controls involuntary bodily functions such as heartbeat and breathing. The autonomic nervous system has two parts that work together and balance each other: the sympathetic and the parasympathetic nervous systems. The sympathetic system dominates during stressful situations and pumps essential hormones into the bloodstream—specifically adrenaline and noradrenaline. The result? Your heart rate quickens, your breathing rate increases, and you become anxious and alert, poised for action.

Once the threat of danger has passed, the parasympathetic nervous system wants to step in. It has a calming effect and dominates during sleep. One of its jobs is to secrete the hormone acetylcholine, which slows the heart and enhances digestion. If you continue to feel (emotionally) stressed, then your body will continue to experience the physical effects of that stress. Are you having trouble sleeping? Are you experiencing stomach distress? Is your blood pressure up? If stress continues to dominate, the parasympathetic nervous system doesn't have much of an opportunity to help you calm down.

A Note of Encouragement

Germs are a fact of life. They've always played a role in human history. Now our world is changing. With international travel and shipping, we're linked more closely to all parts of the globe, exposing us to exotic microbes on a scale that has never occurred before. This is one of the reasons infectious illness is on the rise.

The fact is, we can't get away from germs. However, we can learn to live with them. We can thrive in spite of them by applying some of the practical techniques we've discussed in this book.

There are new problems, but there are also new opportunities. We have a great deal more information and resources at our disposal. As a result, we can be better prepared to protect ourselves and better informed about what we need to do.

This brings us to the all-important question of balance. It's important not to become obsessed with germs. We're not suggesting that you wash your hands 18 times a day. But you can incorporate practical hygiene into your daily routine and that of your children. We want to encourage you to do this in a balanced way, to incorporate it into your life without feeling stressed. Actually, that would be counterproductive. As we mentioned, when the body doesn't shift out of the stress response, immune function can be hampered, so a balanced attitude and lifestyle are important aspects of staying healthy.

This book is intended to provide focused information, to put resources at your disposal. Information overload is always a risk, yet information is still one of our best defenses. We hope we've given you practical strategies you can apply on a daily basis. Stay informed. Keep up with pertinent information. Prioritize what you need to do—do what's most important.

As doctors, a good deal of our work ultimately boils down to two main strategies:

- Remove what is causing or contributing to the problem, such as infection, toxicity, underlying allergies, or chronic stress.
- Provide what is missing or needed—nutrients to repair the body and support the immune system. We also employ herbs and/or medication to fight infection when appropriate.

Using these strategies, we then recommend supplements that support general immune enhancement. When needed, we use herbs and nutrients for their more specific effects—their antiviral, antibacterial, antiparasitic, or antifungal properties.

We prefer to utilize natural herbal and nutritional supplements as much as possible, but utilize medications as needed.

You can develop your own personalized program to fortify your immunity—focusing on either general immune support or on specific strategies against bacteria or viruses. You can also use these immune-building and protective strategies in unfamiliar situations—for example, when you're traveling. More about this approach can be found in the travel and SARS chapters, and additional information is available in the Resources section and on our web site. You'll also find updated tips on building immunity and the latest on emerging infections at www.germsurvivalguide.com.

You can apply the information in this book to augment the efforts you are already making to stay healthy. Our hope is that we've empowered you with practical resources you can use to protect yourself and your family.

Resources

Contacting the Authors

The Center for Progressive Medicine, Pinnacle Place, Suite 224; 10 McKown Road, Albany, NY 12203; phone: (518) 435-0082.

Rhinebeck Health Center, 108 Montgomery Street; Rhinebeck, NY 12572; phone: (845) 876-7082.

Resources and Books about Germs

Brown, Jack. *Don't Touch That Doorknob*. New York: Warner Books, 2001.

Diamond, Jared. *Guns, Germs, and Steel*. New York: W. W. Norton, 1998.

Eberthart-Phillips, Jason. *Outbreak Alert. Responding to the Increasing Threat of Infectious Diseases*. Oakland, CA: New Harbinger Publications, 2000.

Ewald, Paul W. *Plague Time: How Stealth Infections Are Causing Cancers, Heart Disease, and Other Deadly Ailments*. New York: Free Press, 2000.

Garrett, Laurie. *The Coming Plague*. New York: Penguin USA, 1995.

Karlen, Arno. *Man and Microbes: Disease and Plagues in History and Modern Times*. New York: G. P. Putnam's Sons, 1995.

Kolata, Gina. *Flu: The Story of the Great Influenza Pandemic of 1918 and the Search for the Virus That Caused It*. New York: Touchstone Books, 2001.

Tierno, Phillip M., Jr. *The Secret Life of Germs: Observations of a Microbe Hunter*. New York: Pocket Books, 2002.

Publications for Professionals

Centers for Disease Control and Prevention. *Emerging Infectious Diseases* (journal). Web site: www.cdc.gov/ncidod/eid/.

Hurst, Christon J., ed. *Manual of Environmental Microbiology*. Washington, DC: ASM Press, 2002.

Mims, Cedric, and others. *Medical Microbiology*, 2d ed. St. Louis, MO: Mosby, 2002.

Murray, Patrick R., and others. *Medical Microbiology*, 4th ed. St. Louis, MO: Mosby, 2002.

Books about Complementary-Integrative Medicine

Ashford, N. A., and C. S. Miller. *Chemical Exposures: Low Levels and High Stakes*. New York: Van Nostrand Reinhold, 1997.

Bland, Jeffrey. *The 20-Day Rejuvenation Diet Program*. New York: McGraw-Hill/Contemporary Books, 1997.

Bock, Kenneth, and Nellie Sabin. *The Road to Immunity*. New York: Pocket Books, 1997.

Bock, Steven J. *Stay Young the Melatonin Way: The Natural Plan for Better Sex, Better Sleep, Better Health, and Longer Life*. New York: Penguin, USA, 1995.

Bock, Steven, Kenneth Bock, and Nancy Pauline Bruning. *Natural Relief for Your Child's Asthma*. New York: HarperCollins, 1999.

Crook, William. *The Yeast Connection*. New York: Vintage Books, 1986.

Galland, Leo. *Power Healing*, 2d ed. New York: Random House, 1998.

Gittleman, Ann Louise. *Guess What Came to Dinner*. New York: Avery/Penguin Putnam, 1993.

Haas, Elson. *The Staying Healthy Shopper's Guide*. Berkeley, CA: Celestial Arts Press, 1999.

Kabat-Zinn, Jon. *Full Catastrophe Living: Using the Wisdom of Your Body and Mind to Face Stress, Pain, and Illness*. New York: Delta, 1990.

Pizzorno, Joseph, and Michael T. Murray. *Encyclopedia of Natural Medicine*. New York: Prima Publishing, 1998.

Schmidt, Michael, Lendon Smith, and Keith Sehnert. *Beyond Antibiotics*. Emeryville, CA: North Atlantic Books, 1993.

Ullman, Robert, and Judyth Reichenberg-Ullman. *Homeopathic Self-Care: The Quick and Easy Guide for the Whole Family*. New York: Prima Publishing, 1997.

Internet Resources

- Web site for *The Germ Survival Guide*: www.germsurvival guide.com.
- Web site for the medical practices of Drs. Kenneth Bock and Steven Bock: www.rhinebeckhealth.com.
- Center for Science in the Public Interest. Information on preventing food poisoning, reporting on foodborne illness, and other resources. Web site: www.cspinet.org/.
- Centers for Disease Control and Prevention. An exceptional resource, with in-depth information on topics that include insect-borne diseases such as West Nile virus; infections, such as rabies, transmitted by pets; sexually transmitted diseases; and common illnesses. Web site: www.cdc.gov.
- Centers for Disease Control and Prevention. *Morbidity and Mortality Weekly Report*. Data on illness and death by specific disease, with weekly and yearly summaries, and reviews of various topics. Web site: www2.cdc.gov/mmwr/.
- Columbia University, the Rosenthal Center. Complementary and alternative medicine programs in medical schools, herbal medicine links, and other resources. Web site: www.rosenthal.hs. columbia.edu/.
- National Center for Complementary and Alternative Medicine (NCCAM) at the NIH. An extensive site that offers definitions of complementary therapies, reading lists, NCCAM activities, and links to other government health sites. NCCAM Clearinghouse, P.O. Box 8218, Silver Spring, MD 20907-8218; phone (888) 644-6226; web site: www.nccam.nih.gov.

- National Center for Health Statistics. Provides national data about a number of infectious diseases and links to 14 different federal agencies for specific statistics. Web site: www.cdc.gov/ nchswww/.
- National Center for Infectious Diseases. Fact sheets that can be downloaded, links to other resources, and information on travelers' health. Web site: www.cdc.gov/ncidod/.
- National Foundation for Infectious Diseases. General information on infectious diseases and fact sheets on numerous specific diseases. Web site: www.nfid.org/.
- World Health Organization. Web site listing all major online journals: www.who.int/hlt/virtuallibrary/English/fulltextjour.htm.

Information Resources

How to Find More Information on Your Own

Summaries from the medical literature are available online at PubMed. PubMed and Medline, two different online formats of this database, are services of the National Library of Medicine at the National Institutes of Health. Web site: www.nlm.nih.gov/pubmed/.

Patient Information Resources

Several research services are available that will perform research for a fee. Typical fees average $100 although the amount varies with the size of the search. These searches can be quite extensive and often contain full-text articles as well as summaries and other resources.

- The Institute for Health and Healing Library (formerly Planetree Health Resource Center), 2040 Webster Street, San Francisco, CA 94115; phone: (415) 923-3681; email: cpmcihhlib@sutterhealth.org.
- The Health Resource, 933 Faulkner Street, Conway, AR 72032; phone: (800) 949-0090 or (501) 329-5272; email: moreinfo@the healthresource.com; web site: www.thehealthresource.com.
- World Research Foundation, 41 Bell Rock Plaza, Sedona, AZ 86351; phone: (928) 284-3300; email: info@wrf.org.

Referrals to Practitioners

- American Academy of Environmental Medicine, 7701 E. Kellogg, Suite 625, Wichita, KS 67207; phone: (316) 684-5500. Referrals can be requested at referral@aaem.com; a list of practitioners with expertise in environmental medicine is included on the academy's web site at www.aaem.com/.
- American College for the Advancement of Medicine, 23121 Verdugo Drive, Suite 204, Laguna Hills, CA 92653; practitioners with expertise in nutritional, alternative, and integrative medicine. Phone: (800) 532-3688; fax: (949) 455-9679; web site with practitioner list at www.acam.org. To receive a list of practitioners, send a self-addressed envelope with two stamps.
- American Holistic Veterinary Medical Association, 2218 Old Emmorton Road, Bel Air, MD 21015; phone: (410) 569-0795; email: office@ahvma.org; referrals to vets nationwide on the web site at www.ahvma.org.
- Environmental Dental Association, P.O. Box 2184, Rancho Santa Fe, CA 92067; phone: (800) 388-8124. For book orders, call EDA at (619) 586-7626. To receive a list of alternative dentists, send a self-addressed stamped envelope with 55¢ postage, and enclose $3.
- Holistic Dental Association, P.O. Box 5007, Durango, CO 81301; email: hda@frontier.net; information on complementary and alternative dentistry; a list of practitioners is available on the association's web site at www.holisticdental.org/.
- National Center for Homeopathy, 801 N. Fairfax Street, Suite 306, Alexandria, VA 22314; phone: (877) 624-0613 or (703) 548-7790; web site: www.homeopathic.org; publishes a directory of physicians and other practitioners who specialize in homeopathy.

Information on Food and Nutrients

Information Resources

- FDA Consumer Information, phone: (800) 532-4440, (301) 443-1240, or (301) 827-4420.
- FDA Seafood Hotline, phone: (800) FDA-4010 or (202) 205-4314.

- USDA's Meat and Poultry Hotline, phone: (800) 535-4555 or (202) 720-3333.
- Safe Tables Our Priority, P.O. Box 4352, Burlington, VA 05406-4352; hotline: (800)-350-STOP; web site: www.stop-usa.org; an information clearinghouse that provides information for the victims of food-borne illness, as well as consumer education and advocacy.

Nutrients

Most of the nutritional supplements discussed are available from health-food stores, natural health practitioners, catalogs, or online sources. Additional sources include:

- Healthy Companions, a source for specialized nutrient and herbal formulas and immune boosters, including Transfer Factor™, www.healthycompanions.com, (800) 455-0793.
- Health Concerns, a source for Chinese herbal formulas, www.healthconcerns.com, (800) 233-9355.
- Millennium Nutritionals, a source for nutritional supplements and herbs, www.millnut.com (877) 443-1669.
- Heel/BHI, a source for European homeopathic remedies, www.heelbhi.com, (800) 621-7644.
- Healthy Companions Nutritional, phone: (800) 455-0793.

Resources for Water Quality

Selecting the right sources of drinking water for you and your family involves a series of choices and sometimes tradeoffs. It may mean doing some extra research to identify the most important issues and tailoring the solution to your lifestyle and budget.

Testing Tap or Well Water

- Spectrum Laboratories, St. Paul, MN; phone: (800) 447-5221.
- Suburban Water Testing, Temple, PA; phone: (800) 433-6595. Web site: www.h2otestg.com.

Bottled Water and Water Filters

- International Bottled Water Association (IBEW) in Virginia. Bottlers of water must meet certain standards to join the IBEW; phone: (800) 928-3711.

- NSF International, Consumer Affairs Department, Ann Arbor, MI. Consumer guides to water filters and bottled water; phone: (800) 673-6275.
- The Wellness Water Filter—excellent filtration system available in portable, shower, countertop, and comprehensive home unit models (filters to 0.5 microns). Phone (888) 534-8288.
- The Water Store/U.S. Pure Water—national sales and consulting on water filtration and units, including reverse osmosis, ultraviolet, and carbon filtration, as well as shower filters. To order, call (800) 776-7654; web site www.uspurewater.com, or write U.S. Pure Water, 200 Galli Drive, Suite E; Novato, CA 94947.

Information on Municipal and County Water

- County water departments can often provide information on local water quality.
- EPA's Safe Drinking Water Hotline, phone: (800) 426-4791.
- The Environmental Defense Fund posts municipal water ratings from locations across the country on its web site at www.score card.org.
- The Environmental Working Group provides a series of insightful reports and analysis of government test data on water quality nationwide at www.ewg.org.

Resources for Coping with Mold and Airborne Contaminates

- Home testing for molds can be obtained through Prestige Publishing, P.O. Box 3068, Syracuse, NY 13220; phone: (800) 846-6687 or (315) 455-7862; web site: www.prestigepublishing.com.
- Units that purify or "scrub" the air in your home can be purchased through appliance stores or the Internet. Whenever possible, take a look at the equipment at an appliance store before you purchase it. Descriptions of a range of air cleaning units are available on a number of sites, including www.realgoods.com.

Travel Resources

- Centers for Disease Control and Prevention. *Health Information for International Travel*, 2001–2002. CDC: Atlanta, GA, 2001.

- Centers for Disease Control and Prevention. *Summary of Sanitation Inspections of International Cruise Ships* (the Green Sheet). Available online at www.cdc.gov/nceh/vsp or (888) 232-6789.
- Centers for Disease Control and Prevention web site, which posts travel advisories at www.cdc.gov/travel/.

Jones, Nick. *The Rough Guide to Travel Health*. London: Rough Guides, 2001.

Pollard, Andrew J., and David R. Murdoch. *Fast Facts — Travel Medicine*. Oxford: Health Press, 2001.

Wise, Mark. *The Travel Doctor: Your Guide to Staying Healthy While You Travel*. Toronto: Firefly Books, 2002.

Additional Books on Travel Health

American Automobile Association (AAA). *World Passport to Safer Travel*. AAA, 2000.

Hasbrouk, Edward. *Practical Nomad: How to Travel around the World*. Emeryville, CA: Avalon Travel Publishing, 2000.

Johnston, Robert. *Living Overseas: What You Need to Know*. Naples, FL: Living Overseas Books, 2000.

Lorie, Jonathan, ed. *The Traveler's Handbook. The Insider's Guide to World Travel*. Guilford, CT: Globe Pequot Press, 2000.

Notes

Chapter 1

1. Hendrix, Anastasia. Erin Brockovich crusades against mold: State lawmakers told of potential health dangers. *San Francisco Chronicle*, March 8, 2001, pp. A3, A6.
2. Bell, Elizabeth, and Michael Pena. Meningitis fatality frightens Livermore: County rushes to treat teens with antibiotics. *San Francisco Chronicle*, April 18, 2001. Web archive: www.sfgate.com.
3. Altman, Lawrence K. Microbe in salon footbath is suspected in boil outbreak. *New York Times*, April 27, 2001. Web archive: www.nytimes.com.
4. Winter, Greg. Contaminated food makes millions ill despite advances. *New York Times*, March 18, 2001. Web archive: www.nytimes.com.
5. Associated Press. Illness hits hundreds aboard cruise ship. February 2, 2003. http://apnews.excite.com/article/20030202/D7OUIF88o.html.
6. World Health Organization (WHO). *The World Health Report, 1999.* Geneva, Switzerland: WHO, 2000. Web site: www.who.int/whr/en/.
7. Kolata, Gina. *Flu: The Story of the Great Influenza Pandemic of 1918 and the Search for the Virus That Caused It.* New York: Touchstone Books, 2001.

8. Satcher, David. *Addressing Emerging Infectious Disease Threats: A Prevention Strategy for the United States.* Atlanta, GA: Centers for Disease Control and Prevention, 1994. Web site: http://www.cdc.gov/ncidod/publications/eid_plan/preface.htm.

9. Saputo, Len, MD. Written communication. April 2001.

10. W B & A Market Research. *2001 Sleep in America Poll.* Washington, DC: National Sleep Foundation, 2001. Web site: www.sleepfoundation.org.

11. Kripke, D. F., and others. Mortality associated with sleep duration and insomnia. *Archives of General Psychiatry.* 2002, February; 59(2): 131–136.

12. Wilson, Mary E. Travel and the emergence of infectious diseases. *Emerging Infectious Diseases.* 1995, April–June; 1(2).

13. Davis, Jonathan R., and Joshua Lederberg, eds. *Emerging Infectious Diseases from the Global to the Local Perspective: Workshop Summary.* Washington, DC: Institute of Medicine, 2002.

14. Berens, Michael J. Infection epidemic carves deadly path. *Chicago Tribune,* July 21, 2002. Web site: www.chicagotribune.com/news/.

15. CDC. Hospital Infections Program. Unpublished extrapolation from the National Nosocomial Infections Surveillance System. In *Antimicrobial Resistance: Data to Assess Public Health Threat from Resistant Bacteria Are Limited.* Washington, DC: Government Accounting Office, 1999.

16. U.N. sees big rise in AIDS death toll. *New York Times,* Foreign Desk, July 3, 2002, pp. A1, A6.

17. Alameda County [CA] Public Health Department. *Five Leading Causes of Mortality: By Age and Sex—Alameda County 1990–1995.* Web site: www.co.alameda.ca.us/ publichealth/information/charts/leading.htm.

18. Myers, E. R., and others. Mathematical model for the natural history of human papillomavirus infection and cervical carcinogenesis. *American Journal of Epidemiology.* 2000; 151(12): 1158–1171.

19. Meier, C. R., and others. Antibiotics and risk of subsequent first-time acute myocardial infarction. *Journal of the American Medical Association.* 1999, February 3; 281(5): 427–431.

20. Konturek, P. C., and others. Role of gastrin in gastric carcinogenesis in Helicobacter pylori infected humans. *Journal of Physiology and Pharmacology.* 1999; 50(5): 857–873.

21. Scott, Janny. Hospitals can make you sick. *Los Angeles Times,* July 28, 1992, p. 1, pt. A.

22. Berens, Michael J. Infection epidemic carves deadly path.

23. Chen, R. T., C. V. Broome, R. A. Weinstein, and others. Diphtheria in the United States. 1971–81. *American Journal of Public Health.* 1985; 75: 1393–1397.

24. Marcus, Adam. Second "superbug" staph infection appears. *HealthScoutNews,* October 11, 2002. Web site: www1.excite.com/home/health/health_article/0,11720,509609/ 10-11-2002::06:00,00.html.

25. Hoge, C. W., and others. Trends in antibiotic resistance among diarrheal pathogens isolated in Thailand over 15 years. *Clinical Infectious Disease.* 1998; 26: 341–345.

26. Soares, S., and others. Evidence for the introduction of a multiresistant clone of serotype 6B Streptococcus pneumoniae from Spain to Iceland in the late 1980s. *Journal of Infectious Disease.* 1993; 168: 158–163.

27. van der Wouden, E. J., and others. Rapid increase in the prevalence of metronidazole-resistant Helicobacter pylori in the Netherlands. *Emerging Infectious Disease.* 1997; 3: 385–389.

28. Cooper, Mike. Hospital infections, drug resistance rise in U.S. *Reuters,* March 11, 1998.

29. CDC. Four pediatric deaths from community-acquired methicillin-resistant *Staphylococcus aureus*—Minnesota and North Dakota, 1997–1999. *Morbidity and Mortality Weekly Report.* 1999, August 20; 48(32): 707–710.

30. McCaig L. F., and others. Trends in antimicrobial prescribing rates for children and adolescents. *Journal of the American Medical Association.* 2002, June 19; 287(23):3096–3102.

31. Union of Concerned Scientists. www.ucsusa.org/food_and_ environment/antibiotic_resistance/index.cfm Accessed June 2002.

32. Ensmiger, M. E. *The Stockman's Handbook*, 7th ed. Danville, IL: Interstate Publishers, 1992.
33. Union of Concerned Scientists. Web site: www.ucsusa.org.
34. *Antimicrobial Resistance: Data to Assess Public Health Threat from Resistant Bacteria Are Limited*. Washington, DC: Government Accounting Office, 1999.

Chapter 2

1. Majowicz, S. E., and others. Descriptive analysis of endemic cryptosporidiosis cases reported in Ontario, 1996–1997. *Canadian Journal of Public Health*. 2001, January–February; 92(1): 62–66.

Chapter 3

1. Jahnke, Roger. Getting your immune system in shape. In *Boosting Immunity*. Len Saputo, and Nancy Faass, eds., Novato, CA: New World Library, 2002.
2. Murray, Patrick R., and others. *Medical Microbiology*. 4th ed. St. Louis, MO: Mosby, 2002, p. 429.
3. Murray, Patrick R., and others. *Medical Microbiology*, p. 435.
4. Mims, Cedric, and others. *Medical Microbiology*, 2nd ed. St. Louis, MO: Mosby, 2002, p. 23.
5. Strauss, James H., and Ellen G. Strauss. *Viruses and Human Disease*. San Diego, CA: Academic Press, 2002, pp. 248–252.
6. Amin, Omar M. Seasonal prevalence of intestinal parasites in the United States during 2000. *American Journal of Tropical Medicine and Hygiene*. 2002; 66: 799–803.
7. Eisenberg J. N., and others. An analysis of the Milwaukee cryptosporidiosis outbreak based on a dynamic model of the infection process. *Epidemiology*. 1998, May; 9(3): 255–263.
8. Chase, Marilyn. Health Journal. *Wall Street Journal*, April 28, 1997.
9. Murray, Patrick R., and others. *Medical Microbiology*, 2002, p. 72.

10. CNN. Ed McMahon sues over toxic mold in L.A. home. *Reuters*, April 10, 2002. Web site: www.CNN.com.
11. Ponikau, J. U., and others. The diagnosis and incidence of allergic fungal sinusitis. *Mayo Clinic Proceedings*. 1999, September; 74(9): 877–884.
12. Verhoeff A. P., and others. Damp housing and childhood respiratory symptoms: the role of sensitization to dust mites and molds. *American Journal of Epidemiology*. 1995, January 15; 141(2): 103–110.
13. Voute, P. D., and others. Peak-flow variability in asthmatic children is not related to wall-to-wall carpeting in classroom floors. *Allergy*. 1994, October; 49(9): 724–729.
14. CDC. Summary of Notifiable Diseases—United States, 2000. *Morbidity and Mortality Weekly Report*. 2002, June 14; 49(53): 1–102.
15. Murray, Patrick R., and others. *Medical Microbiology*, p. 607.
16. University of California, San Francisco School of Medicine (UCSF). *Emerging Infectious Diseases: Advances in Epidemiology and Prevention*. San Francisco: UCSF, 2002, p. 41.
17. Ibid.
18. Murray, Patrick R., and others. *Medical Microbiology*, 2002, p. 74.
19. Mandell, Gerald L., John E. Bennett, and Raphael Dolin. Chapter 275: Human illness associated with harmful algal blooms. In *Mandell, Douglas, and Bennett's Principles and Practice of Infectious Diseases*, 5th ed. St. Louis, MO: Churchill Livingstone, 2000.

Chapter 4

1. Donley, Nancy. Letter to S.T.O.P. members and friends. *Safe Tables Our Priority*, December 17, 1999. Web site: www.stop-usa.org/news/sbletter.html.
2. Rutala, W. A., and others. Antimicrobial activity of home disinfectants and natural products against potential human pathogens. *Infection Control and Hospital Epidemiology*. 2000, January; 21(1): 33–38.

3. Beuchat, L. R., and others. Development of a proposed standard method for assessing the efficacy of fresh produce sanitizers. *Journal of Food Protection*. 2001, August; 64(8): 1103–1109.

4. Zanini, G. M., and C. Graeff-Teixeira. Inactivation of infective larvae of *Angiostrongylus costaricensis* with short time incubations in 1.5% bleach solution, vinegar or saturated cooking salt solution. *Acta Tropica*. 2001, January 15; 78(1): 17–21.

5. Liao C. H., and G. M. Sapers. Attachment and growth of *Salmonella chester* on apple fruits and in vivo response of attached bacteria to sanitizer treatments. *Journal of Food Protection*. 2000, July; 63(7): 876–883.

6. Gulati B. R., and others. Efficacy of commonly used disinfectants for the inactivation of calicivirus on strawberry, lettuce, and a food-contact surface. *Journal of Food Protection*. 2001, September; 64(9): 1430–1434.

7. Rusin, P., P. Orosz-Coughlin, and C. Gerba. Reduction of faecal coliform, coliform and heterotrophic plate count bacteria in the household kitchen and bathroom by disinfection with hypochlorite [bleach] cleaners. *Journal of Applied Microbiology*. 1998, November; 85(5): 819–828.

8. Rutala, W. A., and others. Antimicrobial activity of home disinfectants and natural products against potential human pathogens. *Infection Control and Hospital Epidemiology*. 2002, January; 21(1): 33–39.

9. Gardner, Amanda. Study: foodborne illnesses deadlier than thought. *HealthScoutNews Reporter*. February 14, 2003. http://www1.excite.com/home/health/health_article/0,11720,5117 69/.

Chapter 5

1. Environmental Working Group. Web site: www.ewg.org. Accessed June 1998 and June 2002.

Chapter 6

1. Verhoeff, A. P., and others. Fungal propagules in house dust. *Allergy.* 1994, August; 49(7): 540–547.

2. Skoutelis, A. T., and others. Hospital carpeting and epidemiology of Clostridium difficile. *American Journal of Infection Control.* 1994, August; 22(4): 212–217.

3. Zock, J. P., and others. Housing characteristics, reported mold exposure, and asthma in the European Community Respiratory Health Survey. *The Journal of Allergy and Clinical Immunology.* 2002, August; 110(2, Pt 1): 285–292.

4. Engelhart, Steffen, and others. Occurrence of toxigenic *Aspergillus versicolor* isolates and Sterigmatocystin in carpet dust from damp indoor environments. *Applied and Environmental Microbiology.* 2002, August; 68(8): 3886–3890.

5. May, Jeffrey C., "Couch potato asthma" and environmental allergens. Nursing Care of Children with Asthma: 1995 Update. March 17, 1995. http://www.cybercom.net/~jmhi/couch.html.

6. de Boer, R., and others. The control of house dust mites in rugs through wet cleaning. *The Journal of Allergy and Clinical Immunology.* 1996, June; 97(6): 1214–1217.

7. Voute, P. D., and others. Peak-flow variability in asthmatic children is not related to wall-to-wall carpeting in classroom floors. *Allergy.* 1994, October; 49(9): 724–729.

8. Rusin, P., and others. Reduction of faecal coliform, coliform and heterotropic plate count bacteria in the household kitchen and bathroom by disinfection with hypochlorite cleaners. *Journal of Applied Microbiology.* 1998, November; 85(5): 819–828.

9. Andersen, B. M., and others. [Floor cleaning methods of patients' room. Effect on bacteria, dirt and particles. Article in Norwegian.] *Tidsskrift for den Norske laegeforening.* 1997, February 28; 117(6): 838–841.

10. Oie, S., and A. Kamiya. Survival of methicillin-resistant Staphylococcus aureua (MRSA) on naturally contaminated dry mops. *The Journal of Hospital Infection.* 1996, October; 34(2): 145–149.

11. Bahannan, S. A., and M. M. Abdel-Salam. An in-vitro study of the effects of various disinfectants on prosthetic and surface materials. *Saudi Medical Journal*. 2002, April; 23(4): 396–399.

12. Dharan, S., and others. Routine disinfection of patients' environmental surfaces. Myth or reality? *Journal of Hospital Infection*. 1999, June; 42(2): 113–117.

13. Ibid.

14. Liu, Y. Y., and others. Acute respiratory distress syndrome following cutaneous exposure to Lysol: A case report. *Zhonghua Yi Xue Za Zhi*. 1999, December; 62(12): 901–906.

15. Rutala, William A., and others. Stability and bactericidal activity of chlorine solutions. *Infection Control and Hospital Epidemiology*. 1998, May; 19(5): 323–327.

16. Centers for Disease Control and Prevention. Web site: www.cdc.gov/ncidod/op/cleaning.htm. Accessed February 11, 2002.

17. Rutala, William A., and others. Stability and bactericidal activity of chlorine solutions.

18. Merriman, E., and others. Toys are a potential source of cross-infection in general practitioners' waiting rooms. *British Journal of General Practice*. 2002, February; 52(475); 138–140.

19. Islam, M. S., and others. Survival of *Shigella dysenteriae* type 1 on fomites. *Journal of Health, Population, and Nutrition*. 2001, September; 19(3): 177–182.

20. McKay, I., and T. A. Gillespie. Bacterial contamination of children's toys used in a general practitioner's surgery. *Scottish Medical Journal*. 2000, February; 45(1): 12–13.

21. Neely, Alice N., and Matthew P. Maley. Survival of enterococci and staphylococci on hospital fabrics and plastic. *Journal of Clinical Microbiology*. 2000, February; 38(2): 724–726.

22. de Andrade, D., and others. [A bacteriological study of hospital beds before and after disinfection with phenolic disinfectant. Article in Spanish.] *Pan American Journal of Public Health*. 2000, March; 7(3): 179–184.

23. Hambraeus, A., and A. S. Malmborg. The influence of different footwear on floor contamination. *Scandinavian Journal of Infectious Diseases*. 1979; 11(3): 243–246.

24. Rusin P., P. Orosz-Coughlin, and C. Gerba. Reduction of faecal coliform, coliform and heterotrophic plate count bacteria in the household kitchen and bathroom by disinfection with hypochlorite [bleach] cleaners. *Journal of Applied Microbiology.* 1998, November; 85(5): 819–828.

25. Sagoo, S. K., and others. Study of cleaning standards and practices in food premises in the United Kingdom. *Communicable Disease and Public Health.* 2003 April; 6(1): 6–17.

26. Holah, J. T., and R. H. Thorpe. Cleanability in relation to bacterial retention on unused and abraded domestic sink materials. *Journal of Applied Bacteriology.* 1990, October; 69(4): 599–608.

27. Rutala, W. A., and others. Antimicrobial activity of home disinfectants and natural products against potential human pathogens. *Infection Control and Hospital Epidemiology.* 2000, January; 21(1): 33–38.

28. Tierno, Phillip M., Jr. *The Secret Life of Germs: Observations of a Microbe Hunter.* New York: Pocket Books, 2002, p. 93.

29. Ibid.

Chapter 8

1. Shiomori, T., and others. Evaluation of bedmaking-related airborne and surface methicillin-resistant Staphylococcus aureus contamination. *Journal of Hospital Infection.* 2002, January; 50(1): 30–35.

2. Rusin P., P. Orosz-Coughlin, and C. Gerba. Reduction of faecal coliform, coliform and heterotrophic plate count bacteria in the household kitchen and bathroom by disinfection with hypochlorite [bleach] cleaners. *Journal of Applied Microbiology.* 1998, November; 85(5): 819–828.

3. CDC. ABC's of Safe and Healthy Child Care. Web site: www.cdc.gov/ncidod/hip/abc/intro.htm. Accessed June 2002.

4. EURODIAB Substudy 2 Study Group. *Diabetologia.* 2000, January; 43(1): 47–53.

5. Akland, G. G., and others. Factors influencing total dietary exposures of young children. *Journal of Exposure Analysis and Environmental Epidemiology*. 2000, November–December; 10(6, Pt 2): 710–722.

6. Bartlett, A. V. Controlled trial of *Giardia lamblia*: Control strategies in day care centers. *American Journal of Public Health*. 1991, October; 81(8): 1001–1006.

7. Novotny, T. E., and others. Prevalence of *Giardia lamblia* and risk factors for infection among children attending day-care facilities in Denver. *Public Health Reports*. 1990, January–February; 105(1): 72–75.

8. Dennis, D. T., and others. Endemic giardiasis in New Hampshire: A case-control study of environmental risks. *Journal of Infectious Diseases*. 1993, June; 167(6): 1391–1395.

9. Kvaerner, K. J., and others. Early acute otitis media and siblings' attendance at nursery. *Archives of Disease in Childhood*. 1996, October; 75(4): 338–341.

10. Ojembarrena Martinez, E., and others. [The role of the day-care nursery and early schooling in the incidence of infectious diseases. Article in Spanish.] *Anales Espanoles de Pediatria*. 1996, July; 45(1): 45–48.

11. Osterholm, M. T., and others. Infectious diseases and child day care. *The Pediatric Infectious Disease Journal*. 1992, August; 11(8 Suppl): S31–41.

12. G. M. Lee. Misconceptions about colds and predictors of health service utilization. *Pediatrics*. 2003, February; 111(2): 231–236.

13. Reves, R. R., and others. Children with trimethoprim- and ampicillin-resistant fecal *Escherichia coli* in day care centers. *Journal of Infectious Diseases*. 1987, November; 156(5) 758–762.

14. Reves, R. R., and others. Risk factors for fecal colonization with trimethoprim-resistant and multiresistant *Escherichia coli* among children in day-care centers in Houston, Texas. *Antimicrobial Agents and Chemotherapy*. 1990, July; 34(7): 1429–1434.

15. White, C. G., and others. Reduction of illness absenteeism in elementary schools using an alcohol-free instant hand sanitizer. *The Journal of School Nursing*. 2001, October; 17(5): 258–265.
16. Master, D., and others. Scheduled hand washing in an elementary school population. *Family Medicine*. 1997, May; 29(5): 336–339.
17. Hadler, S. C., and L. McFarland. Hepatitis in day care centers: epidemiology and prevention. *Review of Infectious Diseases*. 1986, July–August; 8(4): 548–557.
18. Alonso, J. M., and others. Contamination of soils with eggs of Toxacara in a subtropical city in Argentina. *Journal of Helminthology*. 2001, June; 75(2); 165–168.
19. Giacometti, A., and others. Environmental and serological evidence for the presence of toxocariasis in the urban area of Ancona, Italy. *European Journal of Epidemiology*. 2000; 16(11): 1023–1026.
20. Zurawska-Olszewska, J., and G. Misiak. [Preliminary evaluation of biological-sanitary contamination of grass lawns and children's playgrounds in Warsaw in 1991. Article in Polish.] *Medycyna Doswiadczalna i Mikrobiologia*. 1994; 46(1–2): 103–106.
21. Shimizu, T. Prevalence of Toxocara eggs in sandpits in Tokushima city and its outskirts. *The Journal of Veterinary Medical Science*. 1993, October; 55(5): 807–811.
22. Horn, K., and others. [Contamination of public children's playgrounds in Hannover with helminth eggs. Article in German.] *Deutsche Tierarztliche Wochenschrift*. 1990, March; 97(3): 122, 124–125.
23. CDC. Surveillance for waterborne-disease outbreaks—United States, 1999–2000. *Surveillance Summaries*. 2002, November 22; 51(SS08): 1–28. Web site: http://www.cdc.gov/mmwr/preview/mmwrhtml/ss5108al.htm.
24. Tinsley, C., and X. Nassif. Meningococcal pathogenesis: At the boundary between the pre- and post-genomic eras. *Current Opinions in Microbiology*. 2001, February; 4(1): 47–52.
25. Ibid.

26. Berens, Michael J. Infection epidemic carves deadly path. *Chicago Tribune*, July 21, 2002. Web site: www.chicagotribune.com/news/.

27. Neal, K. R., and others. Invasive meningococcal disease among university undergraduates. *Epidemiology and Infection*. 1999, June; 122(3): 351–357.

28. Neal, K. R., and others. Changing carriage rate of *Neisseria meningitidis* among university students during the first week of term: Cross sectional study. *British Medical Journal*. 2000, March 25; 320(7238): 846–849.

29. Robinson, P., and others. Risk-factors for meningococcal disease in Victoria, Australia, in 1997. *Epidemiology and Infection*. 2001, October; 127(2): 261–268.

30. Krizova, P., and B. Kriz. [Factors affecting the occurrence and development of invasive meningococcal disease and development of *Neisseria meningitis* carrier state: Results of a nationwide prospective questionnaire survey of cases and controls. Article in Czech.] *Epidemiologie, Mikrobiologie, Imunologie*. 1999, November; 48(4): 140–152.

Chapter 9

1. Gerba, C., and others. First in-office study dishes the dirt on desks. Web site: http://biz.yahoo.com/iw/020415/040596.htm. Accessed July 2002.

2. Ibid.

3. Reynolds, K. A., P. M. Watt, D. I. Kennedy, and C. P. Gerba. Occurrence of bodily fluid contamination on commonly contacted surfaces and the potential for transfer to the domestic environment. In *Abstracts of the 100th General Meeting of the American Society for Microbiology*. Los Angeles, May 21–25. American Society for Microbiology, Washington, DC. Abstract Q-78.

4. Spitz, Jill Jorden. A hot cuppa bugs. *Contra Costa Times*, April 14, 1998, pp. E1–E2.

5. Reynolds, K. A., P. M. Watt, D. I. Kennedy, and C. P. Gerba. Occurrence of bodily fluid contamination.

6. Rusin, P., S. Maxwell, and C. Gerba. Comparative surface-to-hand and fingertip-to-mouth transfer efficiency of gram-positive bacteria, gram-negative bacteria, and phage. *Journal of Applied Microbiology.* 2002; 93(4): 585–592.
7. Reynolds, K. A., P. M. Watt, D. I. Kennedy, and C. P. Gerba. Occurrence of bodily fluid contamination.
8. On-Site! CBS News 1. Web site: http://www.onsitecleaning.com/news.htm. Accessed June, 2002.
9. Reynolds, K. A., P. M. Watt, D. I. Kennedy, and C. P. Gerba.
10. lifeclinic. Avoiding germs in the gym. Web site: http://www.life-clinic.com/focus/blood/articleView/asp?MessageID=1415; Accessed June 2002.

Chapter 10

1. Schreiber, G. B., and others. The risk of transfusion-transmitted viral infections. *New England Journal of Medicine.* 1996; 334: 1685–1690.
2. Centers for Disease Control and Prevention. Update: Transmission of HIV during invasive dental procedures — Florida. *Morbidity and Mortality Weekly Report.* 1991; 40: 21–27, 33.
3. Gerberding, J. L. Provider-to-patient HIV transmission: How to keep it exceedingly rare. *Annals of Internal Medicine.* 1999; 130: 64–65.
4. Centers for Disease Control and Prevention. HIV transmission in a dialysis center—Colombia, 1991–1993. *Morbidity and Mortality Weekly Report.* 1995; 44: 404–405, 411–412.
5. Berens, Michael J. Infection epidemic carves deadly path. *Chicago Tribune.* July 21, 2002.
6. CDC NNIS System. National Nosocomial Infections Surveillance (NNIS) Report: Data summary from October 1986–April 1997, issued May 1997. *American Journal of Infection Control.* 1997; 25: 477.
7. Vital and Health Statistics. Ambulatory and in-patient procedures in the United States, 1995. *Series 13: Data from the National Health Care Survey,* No. 135, DHHS Publication No.

(PHS) 98-1796. Hyattsville, MD: Centers for Disease Control and Prevention, National Center for Health Statistics, 1998.

8. Kernodle, Douglas S., and Allen B. Kaiser. Figure 308.2, Chapter 308: Postoperative Infections and Antimicrobial Prophylaxis. In *Mandell, Douglas, and Bennett's Principles and Practice of Infectious Diseases*, 5th ed. St. Louis, MO: Churchill Livingstone, 2000.

Chapter 11

1. Enriquez, C., N. Nwachuku, and C. P. Gerba. Direct exposure to animal enteric pathogens. *Review of Environmental Health.* 2001, April–June; 16(2): 117–131.

2. Tan, J. S. Human zoonotic infections transmitted by dogs and cats. *Archives of Internal Medicine.* 1997, September 22; 157(17): 1933–1943.

3. Lynch, Nancy A. Helicobacter pylori and ulcers: A paradigm revised; Web site: http://www.faseb.org/opar/pylori/pylori.html. Accessed May 2002.

4. CDC. Rabies. Web site: www.cdc.gov/ncidod/dvrd/rabies/. Accessed June 2002.

Chapter 12

1. Jones, Nick. *The Rough Guide to Travel Health: Planning Your Trip Worldwide.* London: Rough Guides, 2001.

2. CDC. *Health Information for International Travel, 2001–2002,* p. 171.

3. Ibid., p. 166.

4. Ibid., p. 167.

5. Alonso-Zaldivar, Ricardo. Jetliner air may be hazardous, study says. Strict monitoring program recommended. *Los Angeles Times,* December 7, 2001.

6. Leonhardt, David. Travel Advisory: Correspondent's Report: Crew Members Fault Air Quality on 777's. *New York Times,* October 15, 2000.

7. Pollard, Andrew J., and David R. Murdoch. *Fast Facts—Travel Medicine*. Oxford: Health Press, 2001.
8. CDC. *Health Information for International Travel, 2001–2002*, p. 171.

Chapter 13

1. Lyn, Tan Ee, and Jason Szep. "SARS Spreads in HK; Singapore battles outbreaks." Reuters News April 8, 2003. http://www.reuters.com/news/Article.jhtml;jsessionid=BS3IJNGRGL3FUC RBAEoCFEY?type=healthNews&storyID=2528741.
2. Elegant, Simon. "The breeding grounds." *Time.com*. www.time.com/time/asia/covers/501030407/other_bugs.html. Accessed April 5, 2003.
3. World Health Organization. *Weekly Epidemiological Record*. WHO. No. 12, March 21,2003.
4. Lyn, Tan Ee, and Jason Szep. "Hong Kong seals off apartment block where SARS cases soar." *Reuters: Physicians Online*. March 3, 2003. http://home.po.com/html/reuters/articles/20030331publoo3.shtm.
5. "First SARS case baffles experts." *CNN.com*. April 4, 2003. www.cnn.com/2003/HEALTH/04/04/sars.victim/index.html.
6. Ang, Audra. "WHO experts investigate SARS in China." AP News. *Excite.com*. http://apnews.excite.com/article/20030406/D7Q7N9FOO.html.
7. Erickson, Jim. "Living in a hot zone." *Time.com*. www.time.com/time/asia/covers/501030407/story.html?cnn=yes.
8. Elegant, Simon, "The breeding grounds."
9. World Health Organization. *Weekly Epidemiological Record*. WHO. No. 12, March 21, 2003.
10. White, C. G., and others. "Reduction of illness absenteeism in elementary schools using an alcohol-free instant hand sanitizer." *The Journal of School Nursing*. 2001, October; 17(5): 258–265.

11. Master, D., and others. "Scheduled handwashing in an elementary school population." *Family Medicine*. 1997, May 29(5): 336–339.
12. "Hong Kong physicians use immune therapy to treat SARS victims." *WebMD*. www.medscape.com/viewarticle/451538. Accessed April 4, 2003.

Chapter 14

1. CDC web site: www.bt.cdc.gov/Agent/agentlist.asp.
2. Johns Hopkins web site: www.hopkins-biodefense.org/pages/agents/tocanthrax.html.
3. Mayo Clinic web site: www.mayo.edu/research/vaccine_research_group/trial_297.html

Index

Note: locators in **bold** indicates tables

About the Authors

Kenneth A. Bock, M.D., is cofounder and codirector of both the Rhinebeck Health Center in Rhinebeck, New York, and the Center for Progressive Medicine in Albany, New York. A clinical instructor at Albany Medical College and author of three books, he is the current vice president of the American College for the Advancement of Medicine.

Steven J. Bock, M.D., is a cofounder and codirector of the Rhinebeck Health Center and the Center for Progressive Medicine. He is certified in medical acupuncture and is an instructor at Albany Medical College. Author of three books, he has appeared on *ABC News* and *20/20*.

Nancy Faass, MSW, MPH, is a writer and editor in San Francisco specializing in medicine and health. She is the developer and editor of *Integrating Complementary Medicine*, voted Best Book of 2001 by Doody's Publishing, a literary review service, and coauthor of *Boosting Immunity* (2002).